I SHOULD BE F'N DEAD!

Staying Positive Through a Sh1t Load of Health Challenges

Emmilia O'Sullivan

First published by Ultimate World Publishing 2023
Copyright © 2023 Emmilia O'Sullivan

ISBN

Paperback: 978-1-923123-25-0
Ebook: 978-1-923123-26-7

Emmilia O'Sullivan has asserted her rights under the Copyright, Designs and Patents Act 1988 to be identified as the author of this work. The information in this book is based on the author's experiences and opinions. The publisher specifically disclaims responsibility for any adverse consequences which may result from use of the information contained herein. Permission to use information has been sought by the author. Any breaches will be rectified in further editions of the book.

All rights reserved. No part of this publication may be reproduced, stored in or introduced into a retrieval system, or transmitted in any form, or by any means (electronic, mechanical, photocopying, recording or otherwise) without the prior written permission of the author. Any person who does any unauthorised act in relation to this publication may be liable to criminal prosecution and civil claims for damages. Enquiries should be made through the publisher.

Cover design: Ultimate World Publishing
Layout and typesetting: Ultimate World Publishing
Editor: Victoria Pickens
Cover image copyright: KieferPix-Shutterstock.com

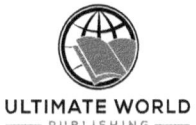

Ultimate World Publishing
Diamond Creek,
Victoria Australia 3089
www.writeabook.com.au

DISCLAIMER/NOTE FROM THE AUTHOR

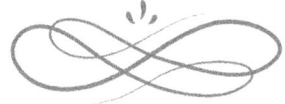

This book is written on my personal experiences, feelings, emotions, thoughts, and memories. None of my medical treatments should be practiced without seeking medical advice first.

Some of the topics/material may be sensitive to the reader and could be triggering.

I respect that people may agree or disagree with my opinion and that is okay.

DEDICATION

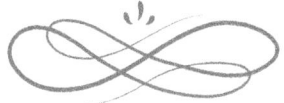

To all the readers that gave this book a chance and
got to the end, thank you.

To anyone dealing with a health challenge,
I hear you, I feel you but I got you!

CONTENTS

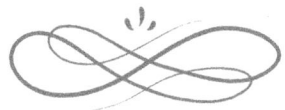

Disclaimer/Note From The Author	iii
Dedication	v
Introduction	1
Chapter 1: The End Before the Beginning	5
Chapter 2: The Hospital Kid	9
Chapter 3: The Bratty Teen Years	17
Chapter 4: My Gift of Life	33
Chapter 5: The Trojan Horse	41
Chapter 6: The Big 'C'	55
Chapter 7: But Wait, There's More!	67
Chapter 8: The Temporary Bliss	75
Chapter 9: Aloha Bitches	87
Chapter 10: Craniotomy 101	95
Chapter 11: The Decisions of Incisions	107
Chapter 12: Like a Phoenix, I Rise	119
Afterword	129
About The Author	133
Speaker Bio	135

INTRODUCTION

Let me introduce myself…..

My name is Emmilia Eleanor O'Sullivan, (née Petdro). I am a thirty-year-old woman who grew up with my parents and younger brother in the Northern suburbs of Melbourne, Victoria, where I still live today with my husband and two dogs.

I attended Apollo Parkways Primary School and Catholic Ladies College, and I furthermore studied at RMIT University.

I have a job and work like everyone else and you will learn that later, although I think it doesn't really matter because I don't let anything in life define me. I am simply Emmilia but you can call me Em.

Define – To state or describe exactly the nature, scope or meaning of an object, something or someone.

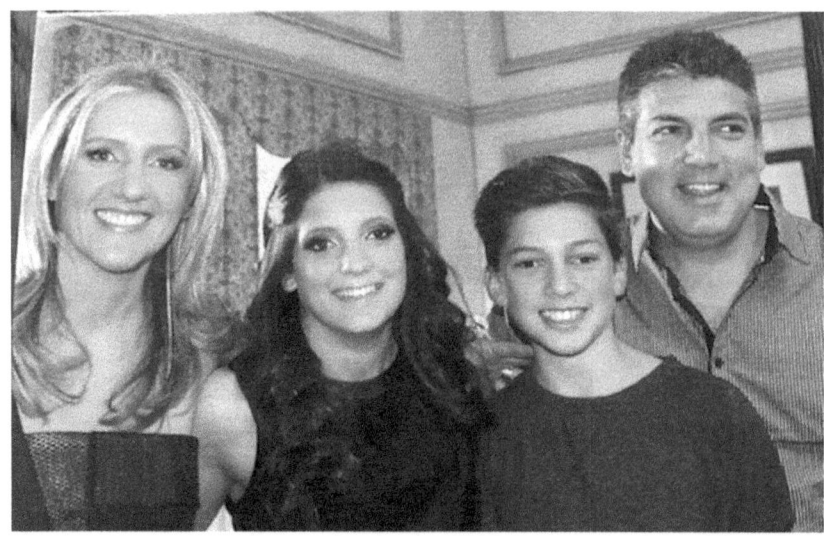

Why did I write this book? I wrote this book to tell you my unique story. My intention is to share my history with other people so they can excel in their own brilliance, in their own way, and to give people their own strength to fight their battles and come out bigger and better at the end. I am living proof of it!

Firstly, I should and would like to thank you for giving me the opportunity to share my life with you and for taking the time to read this book.

I would be so grateful if I could just inspire a handful of people and bring comfort to them with any difficult situation they face.

What you are about to read will be sad, heart wrenching, sorrowful, emotional and painful. Although, I can promise you that it will also be inspiring, motivating and happy. I will do my best to keep you as entertained as possible, as life is not always so serious.

INTRODUCTION

I won't lie to you. You will probably feel every emotion you can think of during this time, but you will feel content because *everything always works out in the end..*

You are about to embark and gain the knowledge about the life of a thirty-year-old woman who has been described as resilient, inspirational, strong, friendly, honest, generous, positive but is also so vulnerable.

CHAPTER 1

THE END BEFORE THE BEGINNING

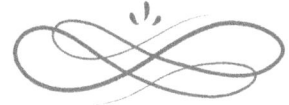

It was November 2022, a month had already passed since joining the thirties club; over a decade of living the adult life. Life was great, for a change! I had just celebrated my thirtieth birthday with the most important friends and family in my life, I was and still am working full time in a job I loved for the first time in my life, which is an admin department manager role for a building inspection company, took a while to obtain and maintain a full time job! I know! My husband and I started a Mechanical Workshop over twelve months ago, more my husband actually, but I am in full support and spend some evenings and weekends there with him. It's so ironic that for years my husband was the one that was financially supporting us as I could not work and now I am the one financially supporting him so he can pursue his dream of owning and operating a business and it feels so good to give back to him. Lastly, we were finally at the stage to take the next step and look into starting a little family of our own.

For the past decade, I had endured so many health challenges and had to battle to survive a number of times, each month and year were full of unknowns. My Husband and I spent the last decade building a life for us, however we always had my health in our subconscious and there was always fear of loosing everything we worked so hard for. Everything in life seemed like it was finally turning around for me for the better, and I was lastly going to move forward in my life until I woke up one Sunday morning—Sunday the 20th of November 2022, to be exact…

My Sunday usually consisted of two completely different things, either relaxing and recuperating from the busy week just past, or the total opposite, which consisted of exploring, discovering new things and getting ready for the week ahead!

This particular Sunday, something just did not feel quite right, it had been awhile since I felt like this but as per usual I just assumed that I was 'run down' because I had just celebrated my thirtieth birthday party and was working so much. I just thought that I needed rest. So, that's exactly what I did on that particular Sunday morning. I woke up, had a shower, and went back to bed to sleep and rest.

Hours went by and my husband (whom you will meet later) spent most of the day outside in the garden, completing yard maintenance. This *never* happens, by the way, so I embraced it. I let him be. Being the kind and caring husband he is, he came to check on me. He woke me up, actually…how dare he interrupt my blissful and deep nap!

Well, what I thought was a half an hour nap, turned out to be most of the day…

It is afternoon when I wake up and try and sit up in bed. I am in a pool of sweat and shivering at the same time. Huh? How does that make sense? I am so thirsty, but don't feel like drinking anything because of how sick I feel. I am confused, very confused. I struggle to take a simple breath, *this should just happen naturally, right?* And I can feel my heart racing so fast that it would beat any race at this stage. I feel dizzy and can't stabilise myself. I put the blood pressure machine cuff on but the machine is not detecting any reading yet.

All these feelings are so familiar, I know them too well, I have been here before and I know what's coming and it scares the shit out of me.

Within minutes of waking up, I tell my husband to get my hospital bag ready and start the car while I use the bathroom as this particular Sunday was going to be a visit to the place I know all too well, my second home, the hospital Emergency Department.

I stand up, take one step and a huge sense of unbalance comes over me, I can't stabilise myself, I am not grounded and feel like I am floating, I straight away sit back down.

First thing I do is look at my husband and say the words I never want to repeat again, "We have to call an ambulance".

The fear on his face is indescribable, he has only ever done this one other time and he could barely do that, I had to take over. He frantically picks up the phone and dials triple zero. Explains everything perfectly to the operator, I was so proud of him, he did it!

Now we wait…

Not long passes when the ambulance arrives. The two officers rush into our bedroom with bags full of medical supplies, a monitor and a stretcher. They assess me, hook me up to a whole bunch of cords, make a few calls on their radio, known as a walkie talkie in Australia. The only word I remember is 'mica', which is short for Mobile Intensive Care Ambulance, which means things are bad and serious in the ambulance/paramedic world. The big guys were being called in, but there were no big guys available at the time.

Everything is a blur, and I have no idea how much time has passed and what is going on.

I do remember asking my husband to pack my laptop so I could work though…talk about priorities.

Then the next thing I know I am on the stretcher and being wheeled out of the house and into the back of an ambulance on my way to the nearest hospital Emergency Department.

CHAPTER 2

THE HOSPITAL KID

Let's go back in time again, all the way back to the 4th of October 1992. We are at the prominent Royal Women's Hospital located in Carlton, Melbourne, Victoria in Australia, and it's about 2am. Most people at this time are in a peaceful state in their home, probably their bedroom, rugged up in bed, where their body is not moving and their mind is in an altered state of consciousness. This is known as sleep, where the body repairs itself and the mind can dream.

A hospital has no sense of time; it's busy, noisy, loud, emotional, active, bright, and sterile but most of all it is awake all the time. So, this brings us to the birth of Emmilia Eleanor Petdro, weighing eight pounds and naturally born at 2am. What should have been the most joyous time of Emmilia's young and first-time parent's life quickly turned into the most frightening time of their life.

They should have been able to hold their first-born daughter and sleep peacefully for the rest of the night knowing their daughter was safe, and would be bringing her home in the coming days.

Instead, they would be rushing their daughter to the renowned Royal Children's Hospital just down the road for further tests to diagnose her with a medical condition that she would live with for the rest of her life. Initially she had fluid in her abdomen which was immediately drained for it to come back again. The first year and a half of this baby's life consisted of various hospital admissions and so many medical tests, different scans and blood tests. There were quite a few hospital admissions due to bladder and kidney infections that required antibiotics through a drip straight into the vein. This was a medical condition with no cure and in time would cause an array of other serious medical challenges for her.

If I was to describe my childhood, I would say it was *complicated*. I did all the usual things a child would do, minus a few things. I mean, by the age of two years old I had already lost my right kidney, it was removed due to it being small and not working properly. *Good*, I say! *I didn't want you in me anyway.*

I obviously don't remember any of it but I have a scar that runs across the side of my right abdomen to prove it. I can only imagine what it was like for my parents, watching me be a pin cushion on a hard hospital bed. Imagine so many strangers staring at me and poking me with their hands and then prodding me with their equipment, whilst I laid there as a baby probably crying and screaming the whole time.

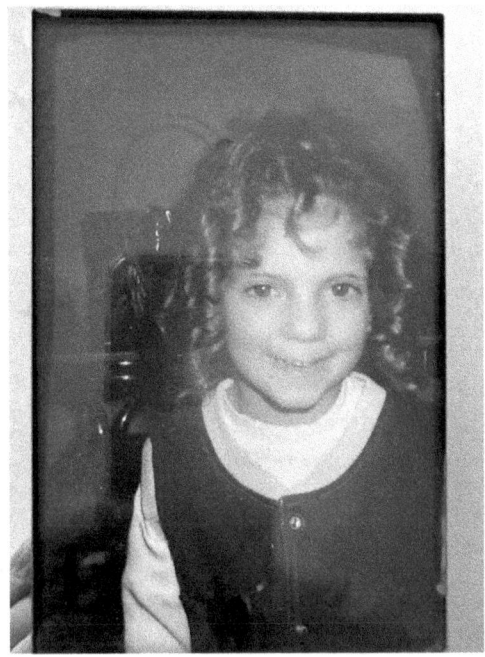

The outcome was my parents being told that I needed a surgery to remove my right kidney otherwise known as a *Nephrectomy*. This is such a major surgery for someone that is so young.

This is the time I was diagnosed with Kidney Disease.

Over the years I spent most of my childhood at the Royal Children's Hospital emergency department and then being admitted on a ward with a drip in my arm for a few days.

I was very prone to infections, bladder infections to be specific, UTI's (Urinary Tract Infections) which would turn into kidney infections, which always required fluids and antibiotics. These were administered most of the time in a hospital for up to a week, which required a drip, needle in my arm, and bound to a small machine that pumped medications and water directly into my veins.

I also suffered Reflux Nephropathy from my bladder to my kidney for years; this is when urine essentially flows from the bladder up to the kidney which in time would slowly scar and damage my one and only kidney.

As a result, my childhood was 'complicated', *that word again.* I was unable to play contact sport because I could not run the risk of seriously injuring my one and only kidney—my only organ that was pumping my blood around my body and cleaning it—so I attended a dancing and singing school instead. I have been told that I was a shy kid and that I was content with just sitting in a spot and occupying myself with something, wasn't fussed over much. I was gentle and never broke anything, probably because I was broken and didn't want things around me to be broken.

My parents decided to enroll me into the Johnny Young Talent Time Dancing and Singing School in the Northern Suburb of Mill Park, Melbourne, Victoria when I was about eight years old.

I loved it, I was about to learn how to dance and sing but I what I didn't know was that it was going to change me, change me in a good way. It was going to boost my confidence so much and I wasn't going to be this shy little kid in the corner anymore. I would attend twice a week after school and would put so much effort in, I won awards at the end of year concerts, and even did private singing lessons for a bit—please don't ask me to sing now though, your ears will hurt. I was a superstar and finally found something that I was good at. I was front and centre on most of the dance routines, too, and I loved getting dressed up and getting my hair and makeup done; there were sparkles everywhere, even in my hair!

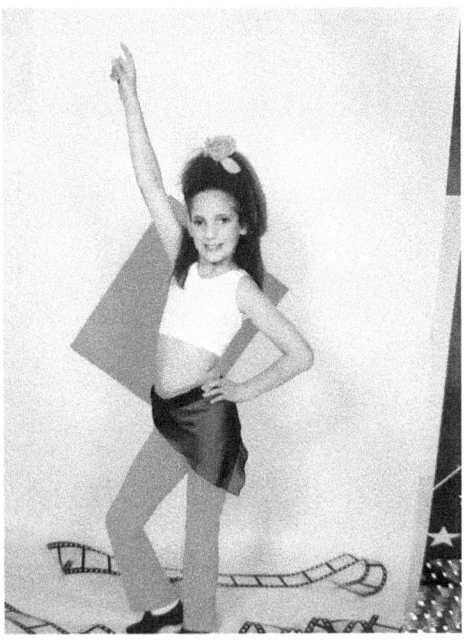

When I was here, I was just a young girl, having a good time with no care in the world. I was even the number one hula hooper at my primary school's end of year concert. I reckon I was spinning it for about fifteen to twenty minutes, but in reality it was probably only five minutes, and I did not drop that hula hoop once!

I couldn't go to sleep overs or school camps for fear of falling ill and required to visit the hospital so I just had to participate in things for a shorter amount of time. This made me feel like I was missing out and that I was different, an outsider. Every other kid around me was allowed to participate in everything and I could not. It was like I was being punished for having a medical issue and I could not do anything about it. It was tough, I literally missed out on most things but embraced what I was 'allowed' to participate in at the time. I had to 'grow up' and be mature at such a young age, and tackle things that no child should have to. I regularly visited the hospital and got poked by needles to complete blood tests. The plus side was that at least I got to eat McDonald's after a hospital visit. These days my treat is KFC, but "shh", don't tell anyone!

For most of my younger life I feared the hospital so much, I never wanted to go and my mum used to always have to bribe me with something to get me to go. Whether that was food or visiting the gift shop. Then Mum and Dad would also promise me that they would watch The Lion King movie that night with me or play Mario Kart on Nintendo 64.

When I was a teenager, I was very confident with going to the hospital, I felt invincible and conquered every procedure with no fear at all. Hospitals and needles became second nature, I knew exactly what was involved and took control of any situation, got it done!

In my adulthood, I now fear the hospital again and I am genuinely scared of pain.

Fear is an emotion that is caused when we are faced with either something dangerous, painful or harmful. I strongly believe this is what caused all of the 'you can't do this' and 'don't do that'. Fear is so influential when it doesn't need to be.

Humans are generally scared of the word fear itself!

Why do we fear so much in life? The unknown? The danger of the task? The consequence of the action?

As soon as we face a problem, it is like our brain suddenly starts to think of the worst case scenarios and solutions to take away this problem.

How about we just breathe, take a step back and assess the situation first. See what we are up against and then come up with a solution instead of running so many possibilities in our heads to just make things worse.

In saying all of this, I still believe that I had a good childhood and that these experiences were teaching me and setting me up for my future and what was about to come.

Things didn't really get serious until I was about sixteen years old. Prior to this, everything was stable and I was just living life with kidney disease by my side.

I even got my first part time job at the local Baker's Delight as I was so keen to start earning my own money.

CHAPTER 3

THE BRATTY TEEN YEARS

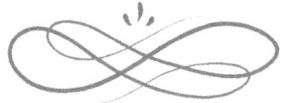

This brings us to high school, as you already know, I attended Catholic Ladies College in Eltham, Melbourne, Victoria. When I found out that I got into an all-girls high school and barely anyone from my primary school was attending, I was upset. It truly felt like it was the end of the world!

I cried and pleaded to my parents for weeks that I didn't want to go. I look back now and think, *'How rude!'* My parents worked their butts off, having three jobs between them and dedicated their whole life to me. They did everything within their power to send me to this school so I could gain an education and I was throwing it back into their faces!

In the end, I loved it and thanked them so much for sending me there; not only did I get a great education, I also gained a great attitude. They always said the real reason for sending me there was so I could become a beautiful lady.

During high school, it was the same old story from my childhood; special meetings with teachers, so many appointments, unable to participate in certain things, *blah, blah, blah.*

The main difference was that I was older and wiser now and I understood everything, I learnt what kidney disease was all about and what I was living with. I knew what the worst case scenario was and what kidney disease could lead to, but it never worried me once.

It did not worry me because I was educated about kidney disease and knew all of the best and worst case scenarios involved so I felt prepared for whatever was to come. It was reassuring to know that there were treatment options and that there is a huge possibility of living a long life with kidney disease as long as you managed it well.

Kidney Disease is a part of me and has been for a very long time.

Most human bodies are typically born with two kidneys. They look like little beans located in your lower back, just below the rib cage. These bean shaped organs have millions of tiny filters that are responsible for filtering the toxins out of your blood. Once these filters are damaged in the kidney, there is no repair and they are damaged forever. This damage causes the blood to not be filtered properly, and this is called kidney disease. Kidney disease has many stages and can either happen very quickly or over a long period of time. Over the years, my kidney disease was very slow to progress and most of the years were just trying to manage the condition and slow the progression as much as we could. I was about fifteen years old when my parents were told there was nothing else that could be done about my kidney disease or reflux and that we would just be waiting for my kidney to fail which would then turn into needing a kidney transplant. And even if I could or would get a kidney transplant, I would be set up for failure again over time as the reflux and infections would just do the same thing again so it would be a vicious cycle.

My parents got fed up with the public health system and the way that they would manage my health and decided to engage in private specialists. Specialist doctors that knew me so well when we visited and could get me into a room in a hospital pronto. We needed a doctor that we could contact directly if there was a problem and a doctor that would not give up and come up with solutions for me.

My parents, Steven and Helen, were also very stubborn and would not accept *no* for an answer, they were motivated more than ever to get the help for their little girl. I am glad they did what they did and all credit goes to them for now.

My younger brother, Jake, who would have been around six or seven at the time was a good distraction for all of us. We are eight years apart and I essentially got to help raise him.

I would and still do anything and everything for him as much as I can. Make sure he was fed, happy and occupied. We used to watch so many kids movies together too.

Mum and Dad worked so many hours to try and survive and give us as much as they could so my brother and I just had eachother.

Although being eight years apart, we have always been close, even though he "complains" about me being a "second" mother to him and that he does not need two!

Nowadays, he rings me all the time for advice!

The two main specialists I had was a Nephrologist who is a specialist that manages kidneys, and an Urologist who is a specialist, usually a surgeon, that manages the bladder. I needed a Nephrologist to manage and check my kidney function, and an Urologist to investigate and see what we could do with my problematic bladder.

At this stage of my life, probably around sixteen, I was currently living with about 30% kidney function, though you wouldn't even know if you saw me! And that's the thing with kidney disease, it's hidden, and you don't really start to present with symptoms until around 10% function.

The first thing was we needed to fix my abnormal bladder before anything else could be done, so that was where we started. It was appointment after appointment with my Urologist, and constant discussions regarding my options. Test after test was performed to check the problem and function of this balloon type organ.

It was discovered that my bladder was very small and was described as an irregular shape. It was lucky to hold 150mls, which was less than one cup of water, before I started suffering reflux nephropathy, which was where the urine travelled back up the tube into the kidney.

My bladder was also "not round" and very out of shape. It was said that it had some major "plumbing" issues and the muscles just would not work, it was an overactive bladder. Calm down Bladder!

Turns out there were no options through the hospital management team previously, however the new private Urologist had other ideas.

I didn't have many options but we had to try all of the non-invasive options first before we went down the track of major surgery. Major surgery you say? I thought we were told that there was not anything that could be done regarding the bladder?

Well, there was and these were the options:

- Bladder Control Patches
- Botox Injections
- Permanent Catheter
- Major Reconstructive Surgery

So, that's exactly what we did, tried everything in order. First were the patches. It was a patch I would have to wear on my stomach close to my bladder, like a big band aid. We were hoping that this was going to calm the bladder down and I wouldn't have to go to the toilet every hour. I wore the patch and changed it accordingly but not much was happening, if anything. Everything stayed the same and I was still experiencing everything exactly the same.

We quickly discovered that this was not going to work so that was out the window.

Next was the Botox Injections, this required sedation and was a small procedure that required the surgeon to inject Botox straight into the muscles of my bladder. So, I could say I had Botox, at such a young age! Anyway, this was hopeful for about two weeks and then we were back at square one again.

Although we were trying to fix the muscles of the bladder, we were still left with the reflux problem so it was onto option three, a permanent catheter. To have a permanent bag strapped to your leg that comes directly from your bladder at the age of sixteen was not ideal at all.

I had to wear specific clothing to hide this bag, nothing too tight so you could see the bulge or nothing too short in summer so you could *physically* see it. I had to ensure it was emptied so I wouldn't run the risk of it leaking. I hid it from everyone around me as I didn't want anyone knowing as I was embarrassed. I was different, it was unusual and yuck!

I had to learn to perform sterile bladder washes all the time to ensure I didn't run the risk of infection. Not to mention the fact that when I found my first teenage boyfriend and did not have a urine bag strapped to my leg and then half way through the relationship, gained a catheter leg bag and had to tell him. It was so embarrassing and thought he would instantly break up with me. It is hard enough having a boyfriend at the age of sixteen, let alone having to deal with something so invasive and not pleasant. Although he did not instantly break up with me, it was safe to say the relationship didn't last much longer after the bag.

There was a purpose to all of this and this was that we learnt that the reflux had stopped as there was a constant flow of urine out of my bladder into the bag. The urine did not have the opportunity to escape up to my kidney. *Hooray!* We finally took a step in the right direction. Except, I didn't want to live like that forever; that was no quality of life, plus it would constantly run the risk of infections as I had a foreign tube inside my body all of the time.

Whilst all this was being discovered, we couldn't forget that my kidney was going to fail and I needed a transplant sometime in the future, so we needed a solid solution. And that brought us to the Major Reconstructive Surgery, also known as a 'bladder augmentation'. The surgery was going to take about eight hours and would involve cutting my bladder in half, opening it up, cutting some of my intestine and using that to make my bladder bigger and rounder. It was amazing what we could do!

However, the catch was that a cuff was going to be inserted to stop my bladder from releasing urine so therefore I would have to use self-intermittent catheters for the rest of my life.

I like to call them 'in out catheters' because that is exactly what they are, you insert a catheter, empty the bladder and then pull it out and throw it in the bin, I was fine with this, it just meant that I had to take a little bag with me to the toilet every time with all of my supplies and had to be so sterile.

The thing is public toilets tend to be not sterile so there was a process to using them for someone like myself. In my little bag, I carried wet wipes I used to wipe the toilet seat down with. I then had to wash my hands thoroughly with soap and water. My little bag also contained hand sanitiser and gloves. After my hands were washed, the hand sanitiser is then applied and then a set of gloves are put on.

I am so worried everytime I have to use a public toilet because I am so prone to infections and will do anything to try and make the environment of a public toilet as sterile as possible.

The alternative is to wait until I get home or a family members house which does not always work because if you gotta go, you gotta go!

This allowed me to use a disabled toilet even though people were visually unable to see why. People stare most of the time when I enter a disabled toilet and there is the odd occasion that someone will say something. It used to affect me to the point that I actually stopped using the disabled toilet which was very difficult and made the process so much harder. I did not want to have to deal with people staring all the time and I did not want to be confronted and then have to justify my reasoning to a stranger. I ignore it these days, though, and now continue to use the disabled toilet. You never know what is going on in someone's life, and there is always a reason for something.

So next time you see me using a disabled toilet, you now know why!

I was all for this extravagant plan but was then reminded that at this stage my kidney function had declined to 20% function, and that the surgery itself would more than likely cause the kidney to fail, so therefore, I would have to have the transplant sooner rather than later.

I was also completing Year 11 at the time, and had my last year of high school coming up after that. So it was back to the drawing board to come up with, yet again, another plan.

This was the plan, I would have the bladder surgery in early 2010, the year I was due to complete Year 12, I would defer that year on the chance that my kidney would fail and would have to face a second major surgery later on that year. Once I was fully recovered, my school decided I could complete Year 12 in 2011 if I wanted too. I wasn't thrilled, but it was what it was and I didn't really have a choice, although I was allowed to attend school during my recovery and got invited to my Year 12 Formal in 2010 so I guess that was a compromise.

Oh and one more thing, I had to have an AV Fistula created so if I went into renal failure, I could receive dialysis easily. An AV Fistula is created by connecting an artery and vein together usually in your arm. This will then grow big and strong which will provide reliable access to blood vessels for dialysis. I had three separate surgeries to create a fistula throughout 2009 and they all clotted up within twenty-four to forty-eight hours. *What a waste of time that was!*

Although, this did cause the doctors to find out that I have a condition called Factor V Leiden which is a clotting issue that basically means I have a slightly increased chance of forming a blood clot.

I do remember one time, I had one created in the morning under an arm block which is when they numb your whole arm and light sedation and got Mum to take me to school that day for the afternoon. *What the?! Who does that?!*

I was also nagging the surgeon throughout the surgery with, "Is it done yet?" and, "Have you cut my arm open yet?" or, "Am I stitched up yet?" I am surprised the surgeon didn't knock me out right there and then!

So as a result of the failed fistulas, if my kidney was going to fail and I required dialysis, then I would need a 'Perma Cath' inserted into my chest as a temporary measure. When a patient undergoes

Dialysis, the medical staff need a really big vein to use so the blood from a human body can enter a Dialysis machine, get filtered and then put back into the human body. If a fistula is unsuccessful, a temporary permacath can be used which is basically two tubes that come out of the side of your chest. These tubes are inserted into one of the main veins and arteries in your heart.

One tube allows the blood to flow out of the human body into the Dialysis Machine and then the other tube allows the clean blood to re enter the body.

A fistula is for life, a permacath may only last 1-2 years.

On the 1st of February 2010, I was seventeen years old and scheduled for major bladder surgery. I hadn't had major surgery since I was two years old and obviously didn't remember any of that! I was admitted to the Austin Hospital in Heidelberg roughly five days prior to surgery. The first day I was only allowed to eat minimal, and then I was put on a liquid diet for another two days, and then was not allowed to consume anything for another two days prior to surgery. It was to clean me right out, and was a horrible experience! I was so hungry and thirsty and was just sitting in a white linen hospital bed, staring at the white hospital walls with a drip in my arm.

This now brings us to surgery day. This was it, I was scheduled to be in theatre for the whole day and it was happening. I met the anesthetist, the anesthetist nurse, then I saw my surgeon. I was going under general anaesthetic, which is when a doctor uses certain medications to make you unconscious and feel nothing during a surgery. I needed to change into a hospital gown and wear those beautiful "undies" that were basically see through paper and way too big for you. *Why even bother with them?*

Picture this, I was sitting on a hospital bed in my surgery gear, wrapped in a blanket just waiting, waiting eagerly to be called and wheeled down to surgery, starving and thirsty. It was finally time. It was my turn, and it all happened so quickly, I transferred to another bed and got wheeled to theatre, the corridors were cold and I could just feel that cold air rushing across my face. The hospital staffs were chatting, and I pass many other patients, wondering why they were there. Thoughts suddenly entered my head and everything just got *real*.

I got to the theatre and there were rules everywhere. Only certain people were allowed to enter, special attire must be worn, and it was so cold because the temperature needed to be controlled to eliminate infections. Everyone looked like frogs in their scrubs, usually blue or green, and they wore funny socks over their shoes. They had gloves over their hands and a funny cap worn on their head, along with a gown/apron.

Then the protocol checks happened, I had to state my name, address and date of birth, my wrist and ankle bands were checked, and checked again, and again. They had to make sure they had the correct person!

This was all done in the waiting bay and then I was swiftly wheeled to the anesthetic room where the freak out happens. A sense of anxiety and fear filled me, and I got scared but I don't know why.

I started to cry and freak out for no reason at all. I had been through this so many times, I knew what was to happen next, I knew I would survive, and I agreed to what was happening. The thought of a mask covering my face to help me breath scareed me so much and I didn't want it, I instantly pushed it away.

They started to inject something to calm me down and relax me, then it suddenly all went away, I was happy and started talking to the medical staff and that was all I remembered.

Next thing I knew, I was waking up in recovery having just participated in a major surgery. What felt like a ten minute nap turned into a eight plus hour surgery that required emergency blood transfusions as I lost so much blood that my heart stopped momentarily, **I COULD HAVE F'N DIED!** The main thing was that I was okay and I got through it, and I was on my road to recovery.

It was day one post-surgery and I was back on the ward now all "drugged up" and comfortable. I had a huge scar from my belly button directly down that is about fifteen centimetres long.

I had a button connected to the drip that I could press for pain, and I turned it into a game as I was so bored.

I pressed the button at exactly five minute intervals to administer quick pain relief. Every time the button was pressed, a small dose of Ketamine—a horse tranquilizer that is used for severe pain in patients in hospital—entered directly into my vein,.

I was warned that I could suffer major hallucinations if I over used it and that was exactly what happened and it was confiscated.

Fun fact, kidney disease patients are not allowed morphine.

I will share with you a couple of my hallucinations that I remember, at the time, I owned a Labrador called Mango and he was my biggest supporter. During this episode of alternative consciousness, I was convinced that I was sitting at my outside dining setting at home and he was next to me on the other chair and we were having a full blown proper conversation.

The other hallucination I clearly remember was that there was a game called World of Warcraft at the time that was well known, the name explains it all, which is a world with characters and weapons and you had to win. Yeah, well, I was a proper character in this game, I was a genuine character and this world was real.

When I told my family and the medical staff these stories, there was no wonder why they took the self-administered pain relief button away from me, their fault for allowing a seventeen-year-old that kind of access.

My mum came to visit me one of the days with my cousin and brother as my grandfather was also in hospital during my surgery and it just so happened to be at the time that the nurse was due to check my dressing and change it. My mum and blood are not friends, seeing blood, especially on her children causes her to loose consciousness and hit the floor.

I was privileged enough to have my own room with my very own bathroom, not that I needed it as I had a catheter in and had to succumb to sponge baths for the first few days but it was a nice feeling having my own space.

So Mum took one look at me and said she needed to use the bathroom and off she went in there. At this time, my dressing was being changed by the nurses and about fifteen minutes had passed so I said something. I asked them to go and check on my mum because I was worried. I got told that everything was okay, and that she would be back.

I constantly repeated myself until someone finally believed me and they open the bathroom door and much to their surprise, there was Mum, on the floor and was sent to Emergency. I didn't want to say it, but I told them so! Now we had a third family member in hospital, and my poor seventeen-year-old cousin became caretaker of my ten-year-old brother, doing the rounds between the family members until another adult family member arrived.

So with a further week in hospital post-surgery, I was on my way home to rest and continue recovering. It would take me a good six weeks to feel normal again, with no pain and the scar had healed up nicely.

I guess I should update you on my kidney function at this stage, it hovered between 15%-20%, it survived, I didn't need the second major Kidney Transplant yet and could just enjoy the fact that the bladder surgery was a success and I didn't have to worry about reflux anymore so I had some time now.

Life was back to normal; my normal, whatever normal is. Hanging out with friends, going to school unofficially, working my part time job. Mum and Dad worked full time so I would help with some laundry, and I loved to cook so I was always happy to make dinner. I begged Dad to take me driving when he got home so I could get my 120 required driving hours when I had my learners permit, previously obtained on my 16th Birthday. I was so excited that day and eagerly waited for dad to get home from work to take me for a drive. He brought me some learner's plates, stuck them on the car, got me in the driver's seat while he was in the passenger seat and said, "Go on, drive, put it in reverse and go down the drive way."

My thoughts were, *sorry, huh? Umm, how?* Somehow I learnt to drive.

There were always two routes, country drive to Kinglake and back or a Freeway Drive to the Melbourne Airport and back, each trip would take about forty five minutes.

I was so determined to get my driver's license on my eighteenth birthday because I wanted my independence, I didn't want to rely on never on time public transport or check to see if Mum or Dad could take me somewhere. It was the only thing going at the time that I had to look forward too. I even purchased my first car at seventeen, a 2004 Holden Astra, it was silver and I was so proud of it. I was super organised so I just wanted to be able to get my license on my birthday and jump in my car and drive anywhere I wanted to with ease.

I probably shouldn't be admitting this but I am going to say that most seventeen years olds experienced this, underage drinking and going to their friends' houses when they had a "free". A free house from parents so we could get away with it.

This particular weekend in June 2010, I met a boy, nothing really happened and I am pretty sure we just said hi and bye to each other but I thought he was cute.

I couldn't even remember his name but since Facebook was around and I am a true Facebook detective also known as "stalker", I went onto some friends profiles until I could find this boy and added him. Determined, I know.

The next day, I receive a notification on my Facebook, "Aaron has posted something on your wall", I clicked it and it read: "Hey, thanks for the add but do I know you?"

Oh my goodness, this feeling of doubt come over me and my heart started racing. My initial thoughts were how embarrassing, you're an idiot, I just added the wrong person and now I have to reply to this random guy and apologise and hopefully he won't think I am crazy.

Then I took a good look at the profile again and released it definitely was the correct person and I simply replied with, "Hey, I met you last night!"

We got talking, we met up again and again, I told him that I didn't want to commit to being in a relationship as I am going to face major surgery and don't want to put anyone through that but was happy to be friends and that maybe we could pursue something after the surgery. My Kidney function was hovering around 18% right now, surely I was going to have this transplant soon.

Look at me being all mature and caring for others. He didn't take no for an answer and on the Saturday night of the 9th of July 2010, we had just been to a friend's birthday celebration and we were walking through the streets and stopped outside the good old local pub and he asked me to be his girlfriend and that was the start of that.

CHAPTER 4

MY GIFT OF LIFE

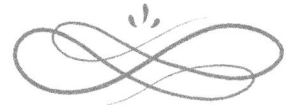

My eighteenth birthday was coming up, I was so happy and excited and I was planning a massive party. I was well and hospital free, and I was in a fresh, new relationship with my slightly older boyfriend (twenty years old). He was someone who cared about me and was not afraid of me or my situation. I was working my part time job and finalising everything to go for my driving license.

The 4th of October 2010, the day I turned eighteen and was completing my driver test to hopefully obtain my license, and that was what I did. I got my license! The first thing I did was jump into my car and drive straight to the nearest McDonalds drive through, and it felt great. In hindsight, I probably should have booked the test for the next day in case I failed the test, which would have ruined the day.

I also had a massive birthday party at my uncle's function centre at the time, over one-hundred friends and family attended, DJ, food galore, lolly table, alcoholic daiquiri machine, I went all out. I am still a sucker when it comes to throwing parties and will use any excuse to have one. The night was great, so great that it was the first time I had thrown up from consuming too much alcohol on the night rider bus on the way home from the city and was kicked off! I promise you, I did try to do something before the vomit all came out but I was too slow. I turned to Aaron, my boyfriend, and said, "If I need to chuck…" You can work out the rest.

While life was happening, I was seeing my Nephrologist every eight weeks, *remember that guy?* He would ensure I completed a blood test before my scheduled appointment and then I would see him for the results. "Kidney function is about the same, hovering around 15%" he told me.

Then it was the routine call to Mum and Dad to tell them everything was the same and stable. I never used to tell them much more than that because I didn't want to worry them or have them ask me too many questions. I just wanted to process the information once and move on with the next day.

This was on repeat for about two and a half years. I graduated high school in 2011 and enrolled into RMIT in 2012 to start my Diploma in Laboratory Technology. My initial thoughts were that I wanted to go straight to University and study Pathology Testing, obviously I didn't get a high enough ATAR score so had to take a pathway via the diploma. I had a real fascination of taking a blood sample, doing something with it and then finding out a result from it that would diagnose someone and then essentially save or ruin their life but at least they would get some sort of answer from it.

So I was going to RMIT and completing my diploma, I was working part time and enjoying myself on weekends with my friends and boyfriend, as well as going to my doctors' appointments. I was even going to the gym! No one would even know that I was living with kidney disease and was at end stage renal failure.

This now brings us to another celebration, another party, this time it was my 21st Birthday. We were in the year of 2013 and I had another massive party at my uncle's reception centre again in October. I attended my usual specialists doctors check up and got told that my kidney function is now sitting around 12% and we need to start thinking about the next plan and the next steps. We needed to plan for dialysis as that could happen at any day now and needed to start organising the kidney transplant surgery.

The thing that I was worried about was how on earth I was going to break this news to my parents because it was going to devastate them. Reality had come, it was here. Something we had been speaking about for years had finally arrived and it was time. The kidney transplant was a real reality now because my native kidney was pretty much failed.

Initially, I told my parents I was fine and that the function was stable and everything was all good, told them this a few times over but I knew I couldn't hide it from them forever. The eight weeks between appointments shortened to every four weeks and we needed to prepare Dad to donate his kidney to me. Also known as a kidney 'work up'. As the kidney transplant was on the cards for a while now, Mum and Dad went through blood group testing years ago where we found out Dad was the best match for me should I require a kidney transplant.

My next step was to break it to my parents and I simply had a casual conversation with them over the phone and told them the kidney function was declining and we needed to see the doctor to discuss a transplant. Well, I was right, Mum was so upset she bursted into tears and Dad didn't say much, and here I was just listening and telling them I was okay and everything would be fine!

I am blood group O, O negative, the universal donor but can only receive O blood and blood products, Dad is also blood group O Negative. Of course I can give to anyone but only receive from a certain blood type, typical! Does not help in this situation at all. Dad underwent all of the testing which consisted of blood tests, scans, more blood tests, counselling, and appointments after appointments. It took a good three to four months before he was finally cleared to give me his Kidney, the gift of life.

I was busy just turning twenty-one, completing my Diploma in Laboratory Technology and becoming a qualified Lab Technician and booked my first overseas holiday to Bali with my boyfriend, Aaron, and his family for new years. Well, my doctor was not happy at all with the trip to Bali but there was no stopping me, I had already missed out on so much in my life and was going to face another major surgery, so I was not going to miss the opportunity to go on my first ever overseas holiday.

I did ensure I was stable enough to go ahead with the holiday and put proper travel insurance in place in case something went horribly wrong. I mean, I was only a six-hour plane ride from Australia, I would be fine. And sure enough, I was fine, more than fine, we had a great time and out of the six adults that were there, I was the only one that didn't get 'Bali Belly' or food poisoning. Probably because I took extra caution while over there, you tend to do this when you are ill.

Transplant year, 2014, was the year I would receive the gift of life; however I would have to jump over a small hurdle first. Towards the start of the year, I had my usual routine kidney doctor's appointment but this was a little different, this was the planning session of how I was going to receive dialysis since I didn't have a working fistula. My kidney function was at about 7% at this stage but was still functioning, *just!* My symptoms included fatigue, loss of appetite, weakness and weight loss but I was still in denial and never believed my kidney had failed. I would need to have a minor surgery to insert a *permacath* into my chest which would act like a port that would be connected to a dialysis machine. This would allow the machine to pump my blood directly out of my body into the machine to be filtered and then directly back into my body.

A dialysis machine is basically a large machine that acts like a kidney by pumping your blood out of your body into an external filter and then pumps the blood back into the body.

This was going to be annoying, not only did I have to attend a dialysis centre for three times a week, I would have tubes coming out of my chest which would be a breeding ground for potential infections and I was not allowed to get it wet in the shower, let alone use a pool. And this was during February, summertime, so it was *hot*! Oh, and I had to go back to wearing certain clothing to hide it again. I would have to wrap plastic around it every day to have a simple shower and would wash my hair on dialysis days so if the dressing did get wet, they could sterilise and change it during one of my sessions. I had to be organised, and this was probably the moment where I learnt that being *organised* was probably the only thing that was going to get me through this.

So I was scheduled for minor surgery to get my friend *Permacath* inserted so I could meet my other lifesaving friend, *Mr Dialysis Machine*. I was going to have to rely on a machine to keep me alive, this was going to be fun. I met the dialysis nurses at the nearest Dialysis Centre to my house at the time and was set a schedule. I was going to be required to attend the centre three times a week for roughly three to four hours at a time, usually every two to three days.

To my surprise, I managed to schedule these sessions alongside my classes at RMIT and my part time work schedule. Oh and I can't forgot my social life, I was still a young adult with a group of friends and a boyfriend and had to do something every single weekend for absolutely no reason at all.

It was a Monday, in the morning, sometime in late February or early March 2014, my first ever dialysis session was scheduled. I drove myself and when I arrived, the first thing I had to do was weigh myself. And I quickly learnt that I had to learn to love the scales because I would be using them at every dialysis session before and after, to check my weight.

It was important to check my weight because fluid retention was the main issue with kidney failure and it was necessary to know how much fluid needed to be removed during my dialysis session.

I walked in and just next to the door was a big scale, I stepped on and I weighed roughly fifty-eight kilograms; so frail, small and no muscles. I sat in a recliner chair and the nurse greeted me before she started doing her thing. She checked the machine and hooked me up to it, then started it slowly. The tubes filled with bright red blood and the clean white filters turned red, and I felt nothing. And so it began, my first ever dialysis session,

I sat in the chair for three hours staring right in front of me, just waiting. I waited for it to be over, get unhooked, stood up, weighed myself again, leave the centre, climb into my car and head home where I quickly change into my work gear and make a twenty minute drive to my part time job like nothing just happened and not realising I just made a big mistake. After a dialysis session, people may experience low blood pressure, nausea and dizziness, but you get used to these pretty quickly and they are not usually an issue. Fluid retention is also an issue. I don't really remember if I was informed about the above side effects, I am sure I would have been but I didn't care to remember them because they were never going to happen to me, or so I thought.

Well, I was almost correct except for one incident after my first ever session, exactly one hour into my work shift. I had been clearly running off adrenaline up until that point, and at this time I was working in a delicatessen where I was serving customers, and I started to feel a bit light headed but brushed it off and kept working. It kept getting worse and worse until I told my co-worker that I needed to sit for five minutes so that's exactly what I did. Sat down, five minutes passed, and then I tried to get back up again but I just could not do it without feeling like I was going to fall over. Now panic started to set in, not because I felt light headed and couldn't stand up, it was because now I would have to tell my co-worker and the on shift manager at the time and was so afraid of disappointing them.

My deli co-worker and I got along great so I thought that I would start with them first, explained that I had just had my first dialysis session and came straight here and now I probably won't be able to finish my shift. My co-worker was so shocked and could not believe what they were hearing! They shared to me they had someone close who had been on dialysis so knew all the nasties and even knew that dialysis can severely lower your blood pressure, especially early on and that I was crazy for even wanting to come to work after my first session!

Yeah, not my best moment but at least that explains why I was feeling so dizzy and so I called my boyfriend and said that he will need to somehow get a lift to my work from his work and drive me home right now. **I COULD HAVE F'N DIED!**

Life continued and I managed to complete my three dialysis sessions a week, attend RMIT four times a week as I was completing my Bachelor of Biomedical Science (Laboratory Medicine), working three to four shifts at my part time job, going to the gym and enjoying my social life. Not to mention my house chores at my parents' house too, how was I even functioning!

This was going to be my life now until Transplant Day and that day was not too far away…

CHAPTER 5

THE TROJAN HORSE

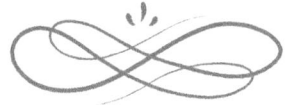

A *dad* for most people is a male role model a child looks up to and loves. My dad is more than that; he is my hero and saviour. Not only did he half create me but he was not going to let me go and was going to actually save my life. My parents didn't have much to give me growing up and that did not matter to me one little bit because I received unconditional love and support from them. That is all I needed and I truly value and appreciate creating memories and being in the moment rather than receiving materialistic or monetary items. He was very willing to selfishly give up a physical part of himself and ultimately give me the gift of life. A kidney, he was going to be my kidney transplant donor and I was going to be the kidney transplant recipient.

I will be forever grateful for this as I know there are many people out there that are not as lucky and have to resort to being put onto the Transplant List, and who knows how long you would be on the list for and when your time would come. You literally have to wait for someone else's life to end which in turn would save your life. Despite the negative events that got me here, I am lucky. I am lucky to be alive and lucky to have this next opportunity of being an organ recipient. If you don't have any objections and want to save a life or many when your time is up on Earth, then please become an organ donor. It's very easy to sign up and you would be saving so many lives.

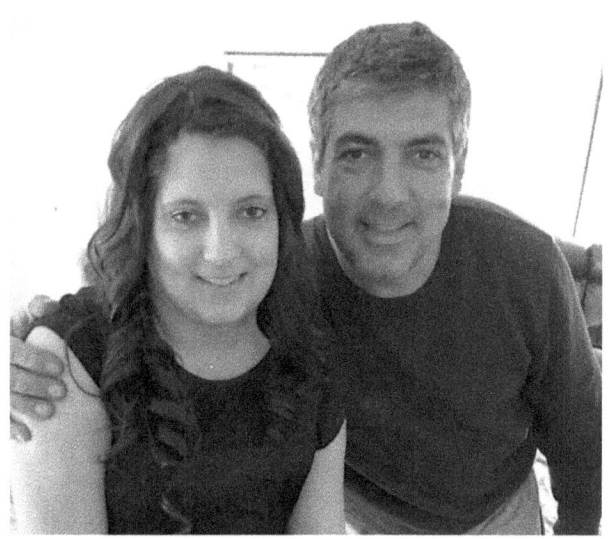

A kidney transplant is when a healthy kidney is taken from another person who is living or deceased, known as a donor, and then that same kidney is then inserted into the recipient who is in kidney failure. And before I continue, I would just like to stress to you that a kidney transplant is not a cure to kidney disease, it a form of treatment and the scariest thing is that no one knows if the treatment will even work or how long the treatment will last if it does work. It can be days, months or years. Every single day there is a sense of doubt in your mind and you ask yourself, is my kidney failing?

Rejection after a transplant is quite common and scary, this is when the body does not accept the new kidney as it views it as a foreign object, so the body's immune system starts to attack the new kidney. There are two type of organ rejection; acute and chronic. Acute rejection happens quickly and most of the time can be reversed. Chronic rejection happens over time and can be hard to treat.

Immunosuppression medication, also known as anti-rejection drugs is something that, at the time of my surgery, I would have to become familiar with and learn to live with for the rest of my life. I would have to religiously take them on a specific time schedule as this was going to be my new life saver. But first, I had to learn how to take a tablet because I sucked at it, so badly. It was terrible and the hardest part out of this whole experience.

Now that all the formal stuff is out the way and you know a little bit about kidney transplantation, I can move on and share with you the events leading up to transplant day, a date that was going to be a celebratory milestone every year.

It took a good three months to prepare for transplant day, countless appointments with the hospital doctors, nurses and surgeons. So many scenarios, plans and education sessions. I was a real information overload.

Can't we just hurry up and complete the surgery so I can go back to university and start living and enjoying my life again? No. First we had to complete so many blood tests, we needed to take enough blood to feed a vampire for an entire month…well, at least that's what it felt like to me. Then, just in case on the very tiny small chance that one test was inconclusive or not correct, more blood was needed to redo all of the tests again. Next was the ultrasound machine, a machine that has the ability to look at my organs, muscles and blood vessels by simply placing a probe (transducer) up against my skin on my abdomen. Let's not forget about that horrible cold sticky gel like substance they squirt on the probe for ease of use. Would be nice if they could warm the gel up at least and then provide a shower to then get rid of it!

Next up was an echocardiogram, an ultrasound of the heart. I always knew that I had a 'good' heart.

They need to make a school for transplant recipients because then I received a big information booklet full of educational material along with what seemed like a workbook. Dad and I even had to attend a seminar lecture at the hospital for a whole day.

Here is a list from what I gained from this day:

- Organ rejection is very common and very bad.
- Infections will be our main worry and can be serious.
- Medication will be your best friend.
- You might go through all of this and still be in the same position that you are currently in and Dad will have one less organ.

So now I was thinking to myself, *is this even really worth it? Yes, don't be silly, of course it is!*

I am a strong believer of everything happens for a reason and every situation good or bad has a purpose. When my dad was a very young boy, in primary school, he was swinging on the monkey bars, like a monkey and had a nasty fall in which he landed on his kidney. Later that night, he experience blood in his urine and was rushed to hospital. It was discovered that he had slightly damaged his kidney and there was mention of it possibly being removed. Turns out this was Dad's left kidney, and guess what? I was going to receive Dad's left kidney. The dud kidney, the damaged one but it did not matter at all because I was very little and he was so big so the kidney was more than enough for me. There was a reason that Dad got to keep his damaged kidney and it was because years later, it was to be donated to his, at the time, non-existent daughter.

Everything was tested and approved for Dad and I to proceed with the transplant and a date was set. The transplant day was the 1st of May 2014. I was twenty-one years old and was excited for this major surgery as it was going to change my life. I was set to receive a new lease on life and it was described to me that I was going to be 'bouncing off the walls' as I was already doing so much in my life.

Dad and I were dropped off at the Austin Hospital in Heidelberg, Melbourne by Mum the day before and were assigned our beds; we were admitted to the same ward, the renal ward, which was Level 7 in the hospital. I had the privilege of a private room to minimise the risks of infections, and Dad was only a short walk up the ward from me. And later on that night, we got to escape the hospital and dine at a nice restaurant nearby with the family, kind of like a last supper, if you will.

Now we eagerly waited. We waited for the morning to arrive and Dad would be first up. At eight o'clock in the morning he was wheeled to theatre and his surgeon would cut four little holes in his abdomen and detach the veins/arteries using tiny little instruments via key hole. The surgeon would then literally reach inside Dad's stomach and pull out the kidney with his hands and immediately place it on ice to be prepared. I think the kidney was out of his body for about thirty to sixty minutes, if that.

I was just next door in another theatre room, probably knocked out lying on the bed at this stage, waiting to receive my new kidney; my gift of life. Most people don't know that a kidney transplant is inserted in the lower abdomen, next to the hip area which may result in a bulge. So now I have a solid lump to the left of my lower stomach area, a little daily reminder that the little bean organ is working hard pumping my blood every day to keep it clean.

You can expect three different outcomes after walking up from kidney surgery. Number one, it was a success and the kidney started working instantly. Number two, the kidney could have gone to sleep and it may take a few weeks to 'wake up' and start working. *Lazy I know, sleeping on the job!* Lastly, number three, the worst outcome, the surgery was a complete fail and the transplant did not work and the organ died.

I woke up and it was option number one, a huge success, such a huge success that it was described to me from the surgeon as 'As soon as I connected the kidney to your bladder, there was instant urine and so we pumped you with two litres within half an hour'.

In other words, they used the drip in my arm and inserted two litres of water directly into my vein within half an hour to feed the new precious kidney.

This was going to give the new kidney the best start in it's new home as water is so important for kidneys.

An enormous feeling of relief flooded me followed by a huge smile and then a look of confusion regarding having two litres of fluid pumped into me within half an hour. Are we only supposed to consume that volume in one day?

It didn't stop there; I was due one litre of fluids through the drip every hour for the rest of the day. This was to ensure that 'we flush the new kidney and keep it going.' I woke up the next morning and I was so blown up that I had put on eight kilograms overnight. I was squishy everywhere and felt so heavy but none of that mattered because I had a working kidney and its function was about 70%, the most I had ever had in my whole entire life!

My first mission since the transplant was the very next morning, less than twelve hours since returning from recovery, was to get out of bed and start walking.

Are you serious? How on earth am I going to do this? I was in so much pain, I felt like I was the size of a whale, I had stiches across my stomach, my scar is a little different and runs directly across my lower left side of my stomach, about 10-15cms. I also had that dreaded catheter bag attached to me and I was expected to just get up and start walking!

"Okay, let's do it!" I said.

The supportive nurse helps me roll from a laying position to a sitting position, carefully making sure that all of my tubes are clear and are not going to get caught on anything. I swing my legs over the bed and sit upright, at this stage I feel like there is a balloon inside my stomach and if I just grab a pin and pop it, everything would release. The bed is lowered so my feet can touch the ground; I raise my leg and place my right foot onto the floor, instant squish. I have never felt this before, it's like I am trying to stabilize on solid water, not that that exists! Left foot is now on the ground and I stand up, success! Now to actually take a step and walk, right foot goes out first and I start to walk very slowly and feel so unstable with all of the extra medical equipment baggage but I am at least doing it. In the last twenty four hours, I had just received a new organ and I am walking, it was like yesterday!

I wanted to walk to Dad and visit him but he was too far away, he was all way down the corridor and I was never going to make it that far even though I thought I could. I also wasn't allowed to leave my private room because then I would be running the risk of catching an unwanted bacterial infection so I was essentially put on hospital arrest. Locked inside a white four walled room with a single bed that contained white linen and I was wearing a white gown. The walls and floors were also white. It was very clinical and sterile, very similar to my experience fifteen to twenty years before this moment in the children's hospital. I often wondered at the time if hospitals would ever change. Transplant patients are not even allowed to have flowers in their room so the nurses station right in front of my room was gifted all of my pretty flowers. At least I could see them!

Transplant recipients typically spend five to seven days in hospital after a transplant, whereas the donor would only spend three to four days in hospital. We would have been at day four post-transplant now and I kept asking Mum about Dad and where he was. Dad was in a lot of pain, so much pain that he slept for three days straight after giving me his special gift. Three days knocked out on pain relief as he could barely move.

How does that work? He has four tiny key hole scars and I have a massive scar but he is in more pain than me? I didn't understand at all. It was day four when I looked outside the door of my room where I saw Dad standing there, dressed in his white hospital gown, holding onto his IV pole, staring and smiling at me. I was so excited and it was at the moment that I just realized that my dad has given me a second chance at life and I was not going to stuff this up.

Let's talk medication and tablets.

Prior to my transplant, I barely took anything, I didn't even take paracetamol for pain. I was too stubborn and always thought that tablets were bad and I didn't need them. Well, now I do, for the rest of my life. I was presented with a folder which had so much information in it, and included a list of my medication. In this folder were fact sheets of every medication and what they were used for, dosage and side effects. Along with this medication textbook, I also received a bright red pill box that had enough space to be loaded up with medication for a whole seven days.

The human body's immune system recognises the kidney transplant or in fact any transplants as a foreign object and sets up a big army to come and destroy it. Pretty cool if you ask me, but not so cool if I need that foreign object. Certain medication called immunosuppressants or anti-rejection drugs are used to calm down the immune system and essentially tell this army to back off and leave it alone. If the medication is not taken, the immune systems army will do its own thing and start attacking again.

So I got reading and learnt about all of the medication and what they were used for as I was going to have to take these tablets for the rest of my kidney transplant living life. First I needed to be put on a steroid. Instantly I thought this was great as this meant that I was going to gain so many muscles and be big and strong, well, I was wrong, so very wrong. This steroid is known as Prednisolone and it is nasty! This steroid is used to treat inflammation and suppress the immune system. The main side effects I suffered was an increase in appetite, weight gain, muscle soreness, bone density loss, and trouble sleeping.

Firstly, I would like to complain about how disgusting the taste of this little white powdery pill is and the fact that I was initially on 40mg so therefore had to consume multiple of these horrid things. Well, with high doses brings potential problems. The tablets come in many different strengths and range from 1mg to 50mg. I do not remember exactly how many of these horrible tablets I had to consume at once but it would have either been 2 X 20mg or 4 X 10mg tablets. The dose changed so often but I can confirm that I am only on one 5mg tablet daily now.

The first potential problem was that I could develop diabetes so guess what? Let's add a sugar reducing tablet to my list of daily pills. Secondly, the steroid fed off my bones so we need to ensure Vitamin D and calcium tablets were added to the list. Thirdly, at such high doses, the acid in my stomach was not going to be able to handle it and my stomach and esophagus was going to hate life, so, you guessed it, another tablet called Pantoprazole added to the list to aid with acid reflux.

Fourth thing; I MUST take the steroid first thing in the morning or else I would be up all night like an owl, and I couldn't even think about trying to fall asleep!

The fifth and worst of them all; weight gain and fluid retention to the point of unrecognisability. My face changed into a "moon" face, I was finding deposits of fat in places around my body that I didn't even know existed like my back and stomach area. I was uncomfortable in my own skin and clothes that I had resorted to the same oversized tracksuit every day to hide it all. I could not even tell you how many times I was asked and still am asked, "When are you due? You must be so excited," all due to my stomach being so extended all of the time. Putting on almost fifteen kilograms in a six month period was horrible and it was at no fault of my own.

So we are up to different five tablets so far.

The next two were anti-rejection drugs called Tacrolimus and Mycophenolate. These are used to suppress the immune system, also known as immunosuppressive medications. One was for the T Cells and the other one was for the B cells. Apparently a human body's immune system has different sections in their army that target different things. I didn't really care too much about this, all I knew was that it was very important to consume both of these tablets twice a day at the exact same time. The only time that I could slightly delay it was when I had to get a blood test to check the anti-rejection level and therefore take the tablet as soon as the blood test was over. It was very important to get a blood test to monitor the levels of the medication so any adjustments could be made.

I was prescribed an antibiotic called Bactrim post-transplant and had to stay on this for twelve months. I suppose it made sense as my immune system was literally wiped out, so something had to fight any nasty bacteria that decided to pay a visit. I was also prescribed an anti-viral called Acyclovir, similar to an antibiotic but aids in the healing of viral infections. Warfarin was another tablet I had to take, this was to thin my blood due to Factor V Leiden. The last thing I wanted or needed was for the vein that was connected to the transplanted kidney to clot up and stop blood flow and therefore kills the kidney. Along with my tablet must haves every day, I also had to keep up with a pain killer regime and ensure I had something to keep my bowels working. It was safe to say that I had now become a skilled drug taker.

Inside my transplant folder was also a booklet of blood test forms and a six week schedule for when I was to return home. When I was discharged and returned home, I was confined to my bedroom, everything had to be disinfected, hands thoroughly washed and sanitised at all times. I was not allowed to leave the house for six weeks and I was only allowed minimal visitors, if that! The only reason I was allowed to leave the house was to get my blood tests and it went like this…

Week one at home, the first seven days – attend the hospital every morning before 8am to get a blood test.

Week two and three at home – attend the hospital every second day before 8am to get a blood test.

Week three and four at home – attend the hospital every third day including the weekend before 8am to get a blood test.

Week five and six at home – attend the hospital twice a week before 8am to get a blood test.

Six weeks post transplant, a blood test would be required weekly until further notice. Regular blood tests are required as this is the only way to identify rejection happening.

These days, I require a blood test every two to three months unless I feel unwell or am admitted to hospital. If rejection can be caught early enough then there is a high chance that it can be treated and reversed.

Human pin cushion can officially be added to my description, by the end of all of the blood tests, my arms and hands were so bruised that I looked like I was self injecting!

Absolutely no driving allowed by dad and I so my beautiful boyfriend Aaron took six weeks off work to be our chauffeurs while mum worked to keep the household going. I F'N survived.

CHAPTER 6

THE BIG 'C'

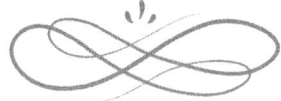

My boyfriend, still Aaron, the one I tried to push away all of those years ago was still around and we had survived the transplant together. We had been dating for over four years at this stage and just placed a deposit on a piece of land so we could build a house together. Shit just got real but what a lovely Christmas present to us it was in December 2014. We chose our house design and now we would just have to work, save, work, save, and look forward to our future together.

My transplant was performing very well and was keeping my blood nice and clean, and in return was keeping myself healthy. My two part time jobs kept me busy and I was finally enjoying my life with my friends and family. My vision for my future life was very clear and I knew exactly what I wanted to achieve.

I was unable to finish my university degree because of my kidney transplant due to one of the core subjects being microbiology and I was not going to risk a semester working with bacteria to pursue a career that I didn't have a passion for in the end. I quickly learnt this when I completed work placement and realised that machines test blood and you are just there to assist and fix the machine when it breaks down. I was already a qualified laboratory technician and I had a new vision in life now which would contain getting married and having children of my own. I always wanted to have my very own family ever since I could remember, so I wasn't *so* career driven. I love taking care of people and ensuring they are comfortable and well fed. Cooking and eating, food in general, are hobbies of mine, and probably why my boyfriend put on twenty kilos in the first four years of our relationship *Whoops*! This vision was within reach and achievable now that I had a working kidney of my own, so in early 2015 I was ready to go the next step and put extra effort into myself and work on my strength which is such an important part of recovery for anything.

Just up the road from Aaron's parents' house at the time was a ladies gym called Infinity 360 so of course I walked in to enquire as it was in a very convenient location, and being a ladies only gym I thought it would help me come to terms with my new whale like moon face appearance. I had a very hard time accepting my new appearance but not because of what I looked like, I couldn't care less about that. It was the judgement I was going to receive from others and what they thought.

People I knew and people in the public, many retails stores would look at me and instantly think there was something wrong with me or I had let myself go because my appearance had drastically changed. Many people would ask if I was pregnant, I even had a few people tell me that they thought I stopped caring for myself as I was in a long term relationship at this stage and had "let go" of my body. As I have said, I, myself do not really care what people think about my appearance, it is more that they assume that I have done something to look this way when I have suffered a serious medical condition and as a result of the medication, my appearance changed, something I am unable to help.

It took a lot of confidence to walk in and introduce myself as the stereotypical appearance of a trainer is perfect, so I was greeted by the owner called Linda and I could not believe what I was hearing. Linda was also a kidney transplant recipient and had a transplant from her mother about twelve months prior to me. I knew straight away I chose the right personal trainer for me and I was actually excited about exercising for once. What are the chances!

Here I was, a fresh year and about to participate in weekly personal training for the first time in my life. Linda would guide me and ensure I would be recovering without causing injury.

A month in and I was feeling really good, I was beginning to gain my strength back and I was excited for my future and what it was going to bring until I developed pain in my left knee.

Originally, it was thought to be an exercise injury, it made sense, I had just started going back to the gym and trying to build strength, I could have very easily injured myself at this point in time. I did the right thing and took a week or two off to rest, hopeful that I would mend from this "minor injury" and then could be back on the road to my long term recovery from my kidney transplant. You know where this is going, knee pain continued and was getting worse to the point that I could barely walk. Sleep deprivation was real too, not only did I have to wake up before 8am every single day to take my medications, I also had to sleep sitting up because when I was lying down, the knee pain was unbearable.

Six weeks of enduring chronic knee pain which consisted of three separate emergency department visits to then be told that it was nothing and to take a strong pain killer and wait for the knee to heal. Multiple ultrasounds, physiotherapy visits and an x-ray to still be told it was nothing and to wait for the knee to heal. It wasn't until I saw my private nephrologist and explained to him what was going on and he picked up that I had mentioned the pain was worse and unbearable when I was lying down. This triggered further investigations in which an urgent MRI (Magnetic Resonance Imaging) was ordered. Within days, I attempted to lay flat on my back for long enough to get some full body images, I only lasted about five or ten minutes before I started screaming the room down. The doctor rang me up when he received the results and advised me to head to Warringal Private Hospital as there was a bed waiting for me there. I knew this was bad and meant either two things, they knew what was going on or further diagnostic tests were required.

I made my way to the hospital and I was settled in my private hospital room, then greeted by a friendly Hematologist who was a specialist who dealt with diseases in the blood. He started to tell me they needed to complete blood tests and biopsies as my full blood count from my initial blood test was off, and the MRI had shown some lesions in places around my body. From my perspective, I was not thinking anything bad at this stage, I actually had a good feeling and a sense of relief came over me because something was actually being investigated and I was due to receive much stronger pain relief so therefore I knew a good night sleep was coming.

A lesion was found in my left groin area and so that would be the first diagnostic test, biopsies of this hard, circular-like structure under my skin. Panic started to set in when I was called to go to the biopsy room because I found out that I would be awake during this procedure, and I had never experienced anything like that before. My name was called and I was wheeled down to an almost operating-like theatre and saw a team of medical staff that looked like frogs in their scrubs and outfits. My attire was that white hospital gown again and nothing else. I was lying flat on a hard table with a sterile green drape across my body. A small hole exposed my groin area and I felt a cold liquid touch the site; the nurse was cleaning it. First, a needle went into the groin and local anesthesia was injected, I scream in pain as the stinging feeling was unbearable. Now I couldn't feel anything so I assumed they had made a slit in my groin to access the solid mass in which they then stuck a much longer needle apparatus into my groin area, then I heard a loud 'click'.

First biopsy done, this same process was repeated two more times to ensure enough tissue sample was collected. The next day would be a bone marrow biopsy to take a sample of the bone marrow. This was performed on the ward, in the hospital bed, again the same stinging local anesthetic is inserted above the buttocks next the hip and then a needle penetrating into the bone until it reaches the marrow. Just imagine a crunching noise and intense pressure.

Biopsy samples were sent off to the laboratory for testing, so now it was a waiting game. And what was only about four days, felt like an eternity. During the waiting time, I was also required to complete a PET scan. A PET scan is a scan that uses a radioactive substance to help diagnose a disease. At this point in time, I thought it was just a scan and had no idea what it was used for or what it was detecting. I was quite naïve about the whole situation and kept reminding myself that the PET Scan is a good thing because we would get to the bottom of it as it would assist and help to confirm the diagnosis. Once we get to the bottom of it, we would know the cause and then I would be back to moving on with my life.

Wednesday the 11th of March 2015, I will never forget that date, it was just after the Labour Day Public Holiday weekend and the results were in. I was greeted by my Hematologist and Nephrologist to give me the verdict. The feelings I was experiencing was that I was finally going to know what was causing this dreaded knee pain and I was finally going to treat it quickly and get back to my life.

The doctors stared at me and gave me the diagnoses, "You have Stage 3 Large Diffuse B Cell Non Hodgkins Lymphoma". This is a type of Non-Hodgkins (blood cancer) that develop in the lymphatic system from the B Cells. The reason for the knee pain was that there was a tumour in my lower back that was pushing on a nerve which was referring to my knee. To my surprise, I didn't react at all, it was like my body had frozen and my brain took about thirty seconds to process what I had just heard and my response was, "Okay, how do we treat it?"

I like to think this was the 'Flight or Fight' response. When we are faced with a dangerous, stressful or frightening event, the mind automatically thinks to either stay and fight or flee from the situation. I was already prepared to stay and fight.

Of course, being a blood cancer, I was just about to embark on a horrendous ride of chemotherapy treatment at the age of twenty-two but at least I had the 'good cancer', or so I was told.

"Sorry, what? The good Cancer?" *I don't want any cancer!* I didn't even know a 'good' cancer existed! Something like three out of four people survive and if you do survive there is a low chance of relapse.

My parents were so upset, crying and acting like it was the end of the world, so I quickly became their rock, their someone to lean on.

People handle things so differently in life when it comes to grief, sadness, burdens or certain events. Some people will embrace it and look for the positive outcome in any situation, some people choose to block it out and never speak about it again.

My parents don't like to talk about what has happened to me in the past as it brings up so many bad memories for them. I do know that they are extremely proud of me for fighting and are very grateful that I am in remission.

In saying this, I am the complete opposite and believe that if I talk about it, I can meet people in similar situations and potentially help someone.

Hang on a second. Shouldn't I be the one the needs comforting?

I found myself telling them that everything was going to be okay and that there was treatment for this and it worked. I didn't even cry about it. I told them that it was nothing to worry about and that once I complete the treatment, I will be on my merry way to continue life cancer free.

I was so certain I had convinced myself there was nothing to worry about and that if I just got through the treatment then I would be fine.

Reality was that I had no idea what the outcome was going to be, all I knew is that I was going to survive this because I was not going to let this kill me, I wanted to live. I was terrified of dying. I could only imagine that Aaron was also petrified, although he never showed it, and if anything he became my rock, even though I stayed so positive throughout my treatment. Now that I look back, overall, I think I handled it very well.

My protocol involved six rounds of R-Chop Chemotherapy. This consisted of an infusion that took almost a full day every three weeks. I had to start immediately, like literally two days after finding out that I was diagnosed. I had a PICC line installed which is like a very long thin tube that is inserted usually into your upper arm and directly into one of the main veins in your chest.

Well, it turned out that chemotherapy stays in your system for a very long time and was acting as an immunosuppression so my kidney was doing great at least and I was stripped of all of my anti-rejection medication except for the steroid.

Two days after receiving the Diagnosis, I was transferred to the world famous Olivia Newton John Cancer Centre to start my first round of Chemotherapy. Definitely not my idea of therapy!

It was called R-CHOP, a combination of four different chemotherapy drugs that are designed to kill all cells, good and bad.

Initially, I was told of all of the potential side effects and symptoms that ranged from increased risk of infection, fluid retention, bruising, nausea, vomiting, hair loss, fatigue, head ache, skin changes, digestion issues, nerve changes, altered blood results, loss of appetite, and the list went on!

Out of all of the side effects listed, the one that worried me the most was the fact that I was going to lose my hair. "Are you serious Emmilia, what is wrong with you?" This was the first question I asked myself with my silly thought. As if hair on your head matters that much? It grows back, it's not the end of the world! However, my biggest fear regarding the hairloss was being judged and looked at in public. If I wore a wig, people were going to know my hair was not perfect. If I work a head scarf, people instantly think 'cancer' or 'medical issue.' I couldn't wear a hat or beanie everyday with no hair, people would question it. Being labelled was my biggest fear, I didn't want the label of 'the girl with cancer!'

I was going to face cancer and chemo like it was nothing, and it was not going to affect me. I would make it part of my normal routine and never think about it when I didn't need to. It was not going to consume me.

After my first round of chemotherapy, about one or so weeks after the session, I ran my fingers through my hair and out came small clumps of hair. My hair was long, brown and thick. I had a lot of it, and it was very much a part of my identity and I enjoyed having long and thick hair. A few days later, more chunks of hair was falling out so I thought that if I got it cut shorter, it wouldn't be so confronting and that's what I did, washed it and cut it shorter but enough to still tie up into a pony tail. I reckon I had my hair tied up, unwashed in a ponytail for another week and tried my very best not to touch my hair/head, didn't brush it and just left it alone like it was a fragile object. Now that I think about it, that is disgusting but all I was doing was holding onto the little hair that was left in the hope that it would stop falling out.

About a week before my next Chemo session, I scheduled a wig lady to come to my house to show me all things wigs so I could have one lined up for when I was going to lose all of my hair.

I tried on all sorts of wigs, long ones, short ones, brown coloured, blonde, different styles. I chose blonde and thought, "I have always wanted to be blonde so this was my opportunity!"

I was using cancer as an opportunity to go blonde, talk about dramatic, I could have just dyed my hair one day but I had to be extra!

I managed to hold onto my little bit of hair until just after receiving my second dose of chemotherapy, then it was bad. So bad that I had started to develop bald patches so I decided to take control, because, you know, I am a control freak and got my Aunty to come over and shave it. If I was going to lose my hair, it was going to be on my terms and when I was ready enough to lose it. Safe to say that as soon as my hair was gone, the wig went straight on. When I left the house, the wig was on, when I was at home, the beanie was on. The only time that I would expose my bald egg shaped head was in the shower and that was it. I felt naked all the time. I never wanted to look at myself and be reminded of being a cancer patient so I had to not 'look' like one.

Half way through my treatment, about three months since starting, I had a PET Scan, this scan was going to determine if the treatment was working. Everything was riding on this scan and the hardest part was the waiting. Waiting for the day of the scan, waiting in the waiting room to be called in for my scan, waiting an hour for the radioactive isotope to activate to have the scan. Waiting in the machine to complete the scan and yep, more waiting, waiting a week to see the doctor for the results. All the while, I just wanted to know if it was all working. Was the treatment working and would it all be worth it? Yes, it was, most of the tumours were shrinking or had disappeared! I felt ecstatic, I was going to be okay and I actually felt good. I had no pain and I was feeling well enough to live my life. Maybe this was the good cancer after all. So now my mind was focused on just getting through the rest of the treatment and moving on with my life.

I got a part time job in a call centre and Aaron and I started to build our house, well we didn't physically do the building, but we were on track to move into our house towards the end of the year. We got a puppy, a blue heeler, and named her Skye. Skye is my cancer dog, and she got and still gets me through everything today. If you were a stranger and took one look at me, you would not even know what I was battling at the time and that was the beauty of it. I strongly believe that my positive mind set at the time played a factor in getting through the cancer treatment and surviving. I would not let my mind think that I was riddled with tumours and that I may not survive. Instead, I told myself every single day that I was going to survive. **I SHOULD BE F'N DEAD!**

That is exactly what I did, survived and after another PET Scan, I was in remission by August 2015 but there was another problem.

CHAPTER 7

BUT WAIT, THERE'S MORE!

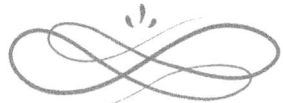

So, that other problem I mentioned earlier, after I found out I was in remission for Lymphoma was just the start of what was about to come for years. Years of pain, torture, heartache, battles, recovery. Medical missions, seeing a glimmer of hope and then taking two steps back.

Thinking I finally made it and was going to be okay, for everything to come crashing down again and starting from square one.

The calm before the storm!

I had just defeated all the tumours throughout my body except for some lesions in my liver, however we knew they weren't

Lymphoma as they appeared different on the scan. The day I went into remission was supposed to be a happy day and was supposed to be the end of a chapter in my life that I was going to put behind me because I didn't want to know about it again.

It came, it was gone and that was the end of that. We will call this day bittersweet. It was sweet that I had just been advised I was free from lymphoma, but bitter in the fact that I was scheduled to have a biopsy to see what was going on with my liver! The waiting game begins again, trying to put my mind at ease but then constantly being reminded I was having a biopsy on some lesions in my liver and had no idea what the future was going to be like.

A few weeks had passed and I had the biopsy under local anesthetic. Again, that horrible stinging solution to numb the area and a really long biopsy needle inserted straight into the middle of my abdomen next to my rib cage and *Click*! That loud noise that lets us know the biopsy needle had taken a tiny tissue sample from my liver. Three tissue samples to be exact. Again, more waiting, this time we had to wait a couple of weeks for the laboratory to test the sample before I got the results…

Epstein Barr Virus Smooth Muscle Tumours, which are extremely rare.

A secondary cancer, but this one was not your typical cancer. These tumours were extremely slow growing and do not spread via the blood stream. Oh not to mention the fact that no doctor in Victoria or Australia had ever heard of these tumours, let alone know how to treat them. Not even the Peter McCallum Cancer Hospital! A hospital that had been around for so many years and was an expert at treating cancer! At least I knew they weren't going to spread via the blood stream to my other organs, sort of. You have got to take the positives out of a bad situation, right? As they were slow growing and were not going to spread, we had time with this one. This was very unusual for me, I didn't know how to react, feel, or even think. Usually I would receive a diagnosis, work out a treatment plan with the doctor, complete the treatment plan and move on to continue my life.

So many questions and scenarios ran through my head: What do I do now? Are they going to attempt to treat them? Will I survive? Surely we could just surgically remove them? What if I did more Chemotherapy? Radiation? Are these tumours going to take over my body? Is this it? How will we treat these without a treatment plan? How can I live with cancer? I want to get married and have kids, how will this happen? My parents and husband! How will they cope with this? How will I tell them? I can't leave them, I am too young, I am not ready to leave this planet!

So I was told by my doctor at the time that they would be conducting some research as they did find a couple of research papers from America with these types of cancer and I would see them in a few weeks. So my husband and I also did our own 'research,' also known as *Dr Google*. Probably the single worst possible thing anyone can ever do especially when the word cancer is involved. Thinking this would ease my mind, it ended up making me more confused and scared than ever! Although I am still a culprit today, please do not use Dr Google! *I really need to take my own advice.*

Basically, we didn't find much initially as suspected, other than the words 'life threatening', 'death' and 'survival statistics'. Let's talk stats for a minute; while they are somewhat useful and bring insight into any situation, I believe medical stats are scary and untrue. I am living proof that stats can be untrue so do not get so caught up on them. If we were to believe the stats, they suggest that I should not be here living on this earth.

After a few appointments, the oncologist did their own research and discovered the Chemotherapy was not going to be effective as the tumours were slow growing plus I had just finished a cycle of intense chemotherapy. So they discovered a treatment called SIRT, an internal radiation. Surgery was also not an option because there were so many tiny tumours that they would have to basically remove the liver and give me a new one, which was something I did not want!

Why wouldn't I want a new organ that was going to fix this issue? Because if I was to receive another transplant, I would have to go on a large amount of anti rejection medication again which would be a huge risk. An incredible risk of relapsing and having to battle Lymphoma again.

Basically, the procedure involved directly inserting radiation beads into the tumours of my liver via the main vein in my groin, all under local anesthetic. The idea was that the radiation would kill off most of the tumours in the liver. As it turned out, the doctors advised that I received a 'mixed response' from this treatment itself. Some tumours remained the same, some become inactive and a couple shrunk, none of them disappeared.

I was also required to have six-monthly Pet Scans to monitor the progress of the disease. *Disease*, it's such a horrible word, reminds me that there is something wrong with me.

At my next scan result consultation, I was told there were more tiny little tumours all over the liver and one tumour on the left side of my neck. Upon investigation, I could feel the one in my neck, it was very small and hard, painful to touch, and less than 1cm. It didn't really worry me at this stage as you wouldn't even know it was there, and completely forgot about it most of the time. But of course, I would undergo another biopsy under local anesthetic, this time on my neck to verify that it was a smooth muscle tumour and yes it was!

So, I was back on watch and wait for a while until the doctors could research and come up with another idea. This time it was a medication called *Everolimus* which is an immunosuppressant. This drug was in the anti-rejection drug family but there were studies that suggested it would have the ability to fight off tumours, these are called mTOR inhibitors to be exact.

I had to be on high doses of this medication which came with great side effects and I got most of them. These side effects included bloating, nausea, stomach upset, pain in muscles, cough, infections, fatigue, and the tumours were growing.

I was also experiencing a lot of infections and my scans were showing that the disease was progressing. More tumours were appearing and the existing ones started to grow. I was constantly in and out of hospital treating infections with IV antibiotics. And at this stage, I had the smooth muscle tumours in my liver, neck, groin and who knows where else! I had to put a stop to it and pleaded with my medical team to take me off *Everolimus* or reduce it at least. The biggest worry was that because I was not on any immunosuppression except the *Everolimus* and the Prednisolone, the doctors were worried about losing the kidney.

I was also worried about loosing the kidney but I did not feel comfortable with tumours growing in my body either so I had to take the risk. My thoughts were that if the kidney was not to survive, there was always dialysis. If the tumours overtook my body, there was no chance of survival.

At the time I was getting blood tests every three to four weeks to monitor my kidney function and I had so many different doses and strengths of *Everolimus* at home from the dose being adjusted all the time, so I decided to start lowering the dose myself. Very slowly and very slightly.

For example I was on 2mg twice a day so I lowered it to 1.5mg at night for a week or two then had my blood test and continued to lower the dose every 2 weeks by 0.5mg and then 0.25mg until I was on 0.75mg twice a day.

Continued to receive blood tests and my kidney function was perfect and I was starting to feel good as the side effects were being reduced.

This went on for a few months without the doctors knowing and I can't stress to you enough that this was a huge risk I was taking so please do not try this on your own.

For me it was about life or death and I was prepared to sacrifice the kidney to preserve my life and control the tumours.

This brings us towards the end of 2016 so I have lived with the tumours for over one year at this stage and my main concern at this stage is that the tumours were going to keep growing and appearing and that was it, my life was going to end. The word *terminal* was even mentioned and that destroyed me. Terminal is the end of something so I was told that my life could end and I never want to hear that word again. I spent a whole week in bed not knowing what to do with myself, I almost gave up. **I WAS GOING TO F'N DIE!**

I was scheduled for another appointment with the oncologist and they had found a promising therapy that was used in America which suggested that this therapy could essentially fight off the tumours or at least what was causing them. It is called Cytotoxic Targeted T Cell Therapy which is an immunotherapy that teaches your own immune cells to be better and attach things like cancer and disease.

From multiple pathology tissue tests from my various biopsies, we have learnt the following about the tumours/cancer:

1. They are slow growing.
2. They do not spread via the blood stream.
3. Each new tumour is a new occurrence.
4. The human bodies immune system, in particular T Cells were responsible for fighting off the EBV Virus and therefore if that virus was inactive, the tumours would then shrink and become inactive.

Great! I now was feeling like a guinea pig and everything was being thrown at me to 'see if it would work'.

Well, I went through a few rounds of T Cell Therapy, felt a little special as these cells were being flown into Australia all the way from the USA, just for me!

The results, inconclusive, the tumours did not disappear nor did they grow or get worse so I guess that was a win right?

At this stage, if the tumours were stable, as in, if they were the same as my last scan and not causing any issues, then I was happy. They could just live there and I could just live my life as I had so many plans for my future!

CHAPTER 8

THE TEMPORARY BLISS

Before I continue to tell you how great my life would become in 2017, or thought it was going to be anyway, I would like to share a little story that occurred in the middle of 2016.

I was at a routine appointment and my blood pressure and heart rate were tested as per usual, but this time my heart rate was up there around the 140 beats per minute, when the range should be between 60-90, so this was not good. It was a Friday morning and I knew exactly what was to come, I was going to be asked to present to the emergency department for further testing and will most likely be admitted, just what I wanted to do before a weekend. So being the good little patient that I was, I did the right thing and went in. Some testing was done which involved scans and a specific scan to test for blood clots as I had the symptoms and the Factor V Leiden so I was at an increased risk.

It was discovered that I had a blood clot in my lung, throw an infection in there too and to top it all off, I was scheduled to jump on a plane to Thailand ten days later to attend a wedding. So the routine IV antibiotics in hospital along with the blood thinning medication and I was on that plane to Thailand. The trip was planned for so long and I was so determined to not miss it that I did everything within my power to go on that holiday, and I did!

Anyway, let's get back to my life, it's the start of 2017, tumours were still stable, Aaron and I were living in our own newly built house for over a year now, being adults. I was working and as healthy as I could be, life was great! At this stage, Aaron and I had been together for seven years now and I really wanted to move onto the next chapter in my life and thought that it was the perfect timing. Me being the controlling organiser of our relationship and Aaron being the indecisive one, I had organised a meeting with a jeweler from Sydney, he was a friend of my uncle's and he was in Melbourne at the time. He designed my engagement ring with the deal that Aaron and I would have to go to Sydney and retrieve the ring one day. I know, call me crazy for designing and ordering my engagement ring without a proper proposal but I think at this stage, it was inevitable that we would get married. Our plan was to always build our house first and then get married.

We were both working like crazy and had no idea when we would even find the time or money to head to Sydney to pick up the ring so it was forgotten about for a while except sneaky little Aaron had a different plan that I had no idea about! Aaron's best friend had recently moved to Sydney temporarily and visited Melbourne quite frequently, so he brought the precious goods down to Melbourne one time and they hid the ring under our chest of drawers in the bedroom.

The 14th of February 2017, Valentine's Day, Aaron had organised the day off work which was very strange because we do not celebrate Valentine's Day at all and never have since this exact date in 2017. We believe that we don't need a specific day to celebrate our love because we can do that every day! *Aww, yuck!* All I was told was to take the day off and to not plan anything as we had to be up at 3am, and I had to wear something warm. *What the...?*

I didn't question it, I embraced it because for once he was organising everything and I just had to listen and follow instructions. So we were up at 3am and out the door by 3:30am, and I had no idea where we were going or what he had planned, all I knew was that the morning was fresh and we were heading somewhere out the Yarra Valley Way.

On the way, it started to rain, very lightly, spitting to be exact and I noticed this nervousness come from Aaron but it didn't last long so I thought nothing of it. Still dark, probably around 5am now and we arrived at this beautiful resort, so I instantly thought we were going to have a beautiful early breakfast and participate in various activities at the hotel/resort for the day. We were sitting in the foyer and random people started to arrive, again being Valentine's day, I just thought it was extra busy for the day then our names were called up to go to the front desk. Confused look on my face, I look at Aaron and proceed to walk up to the desk with him, we are greeted by a male with a piece of paper in his hand. He started to explain things about safety and requires us to sign a consent form. I have finally just realised that Aaron has organised for us to go on a hot air balloon, my number one thing that I had always wanted to do.

What a great surprise! I was so excited and everything started to make sense now, the early morning wake up because we needed to be on time as we only had a very tight window to take off. Timing was everything as the balloon was guided by the wind. The rain, obviously the whole experience was cancelled if it rains. So now, we tested and prepped for the hot air balloon flight. The operator performed wind tests and picked the best spot to take off, the timing was set perfectly and our landing spot was determined. Everyone joined in to help unpack the balloon and set it up, fire started and soon enough the flight was ready. We took off just as the sun started to rise and it was the single most magical thing I had experienced. The gliding feeling in the sky, taking in all the beautiful scenery, and literally not one worry in my mind.

It's a different world up there and the feeling is inexpressible. It is seriously a must thing to do!

So we were in the air and I was having the best time ever and thinking that this was the best thing to happen in my life at that moment. *What more could I ask for?* I thought, but it got better. Aaron pulled a ring out of his jacket pocket and simply says, "Emmilia, will you marry me?"

My first response, and initial thoughts was, "Umm, isn't that ring supposed to be in Sydney?"

Seriously Emmilia, way to ruin the moment! It was quickly followed with the biggest smile ever and an, "Of course!"

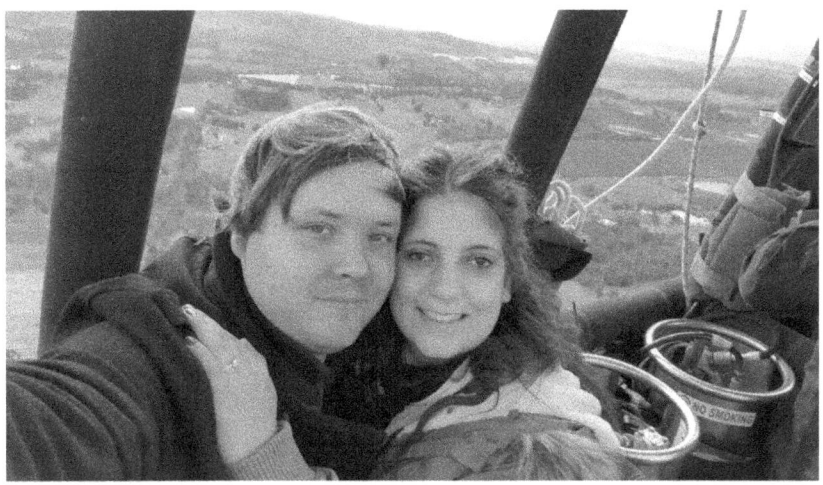

Then I got a champagne breakfast afterwards so I was sort of right with what I initially thought we were going to do.

Life was great at the moment. I was freshly engaged to my teenage sweet heart and it was now March 2017 and we were boarding a flight to Sri Lanka with some friends. We never thought that we would go to Sri Lanka, however we had this great opportunity presented to us to go with my high school friend and her partner as he was from there so we thought *why not*! We did all sorts of things while we were over there, but I remember one particular day where we climbed Lion Rock also known as *Sigiriya*. And this was where I really learnt my fitness levels were not great, but I still powered through the heat and stairs and got to the Lions Feet, which was probably 75% up. I was proud and felt that I accomplished something with the help of my fiancé.

We arrived back in Melbourne a week before our engagement party, can you believe we chose Saturday the 1st of April 2017 to celebrate out engagement, what a joke! A massive party with all of our family and friends and we were excited as we had our wedding booked for Saturday the 17th of February 2018. Like I said before; life was great and we had so much to look forward to. I was finally in a place where I thought I was able to move on from the past few years and live my life…until a week after the party.

I was rushed to the Royal Melbourne Hospital, this time by my parents, with severe pain on the side of my left chest along with trouble breathing. Every breath I took was accompanied by excruciating pain. And this pain was next level; I had never felt pain like this before and never want to feel it again. The pain and vision will never leave my mind and I still remember today what this pain felt like. Imagine sharp razor blades digging into your lung via the side of your chest through your rib cage, and feeling too scared to inhale as you knew the pain would come and you would scream.

In the emergency hospital bed, I had told my parents to leave as it was getting late and they had work the next day. As usual, I reassured them I would be fine and I would update them when I was on the ward. I would also be calling Aaron for a bit so he would distract me.

That's exactly what I did, called Aaron and let out the biggest scream and explained to him that I was in so much pain and was waiting for the nurses and doctors to provide me with pain relief.

Aaron describes this call as frightening; he honestly thought that I thought I was dying and he was genuinely scared, I was also scared. This phone call to Aaron was so scary he had to pull over and recover from an anxiety attack himself as he was scared for his future wife's life. This also caused him to have flashbacks & panic attacks, similar to that of PTSD for a long time.

It was overcome with time and being exposed to the medical world, Aaron essentially grew thick skin and learnt to overcome the fear.

It was a long night, and I was admitted to the Peter McCallum Cancer Hospital right next door as I was a patient of theirs, put on heavy pain medication and slept most of the night. Aaron was lucky enough to spend the night with me in my own private room! Morning came and my pain was somewhat under control but my breathing was not great. I could barely breathe, and the breaths I was able to take were quick and sharp, with lots of little breaths. My heart rate was elevated and my blood pressure was low. Countless MET calls which stands for Medical Emergency Team and is a specialised team of doctors and nurses which respond immediately to a call for urgent medical help. This would be a first time experience for me, the nurse warns myself and anyone else in the room that an announcement is going to go out to a team of highly experienced doctors and nurses, usually ICU and Emergency types. So many doctors were going to come rushing in and start assessing me, it was very confronting. Every single time this was done, I was conscious and fine so the MET call criteria was altered so I could have some peace.

Still not knowing what was wrong, I had to par-take in a procedure called a *Bronchoscopy* to see if it would help diagnose the issue or at least give us a clue. Basically, they put a tube down your throat while you are asleep to see inside your lungs for any abnormalities. Yep, you guessed it! Another Smooth Muscle Tumour which caused Pneumonia. The next day, I was scheduled for another Bronchoscopy to remove the tumour via laser and was put on heavy antibiotics to treat the Pneumonia. **HOW AM I NOT F'N DEAD!**

Once the tumour was removed, I also had to complete five rounds of radiation therapy which was when beams of instense energy were used to kill off cancer cells.

It did not stop there! Later on in 2017, I started to get UTI's and bladder infections, I was in and out of hospital on a monthly basis and then endured my first ever experience of *Urosepsis*. Urosepsis is an infection that starts in the bladder and enters the blood stream. When you experience urosepsis, it happens so quickly and you decline rapidly, sometime in minutes. Your heart rate increases and you can feel it, blood pressure drops and you feel dizzy. You are unable to consume food or water, and if you do it just comes straight back out again. The outcome of sepsis is an Intensive Care Unit admission in the hospital, however I recovered so quickly I was discharged directly from ICU, something that never happens!

Not long after, I experienced another ICU sepsis admission, but this time I was induced in a three day coma as sepsis starts to shut down all of the organs in the human body. A medically induced coma is used in these types of situations to help prevent and preserve organ function. I obviously survived it with no damage done to my organs thankfully as the coma is not guaranteed to save the organs or the brain. **I COULD BE F'N DEAD!**

We are in November 2017 now and I had to have a cystoscopy. This was to look inside my bladder this time to check for anything that was not supposed to be there using a camera and thin tube. I will give you one guess? Yep, another Smooth Muscle Tumour on the inside of my bladder that was causing a build up of bacteria which of course was causing the infections every month.

You may be wondering why I had all these other tumours appear when I was told that everything was stable...well, it turned out that the regular PET Scans failed to pick up on some of the tumours and of course we did not know they were there until they started to cause an issue. So most of the Bladder Tumour was zapped with a laser and I was suddenly okay again, which was perfect timing as I had to attend my wedding in about three months and I was not going to miss that!

While all of these medical episodes kept happening, wedding planning was in full swing. We had ten months to plan our wedding and it was the best time ever. I love any excuse for a celebration or party and I was organising the biggest party of my life. First thing that needed to be secured was the venue. I looked up a few online, visited Potters Receptions in Warrandyte on a weekend, and loved it so much that a wedding date and venue was booked on the spot.

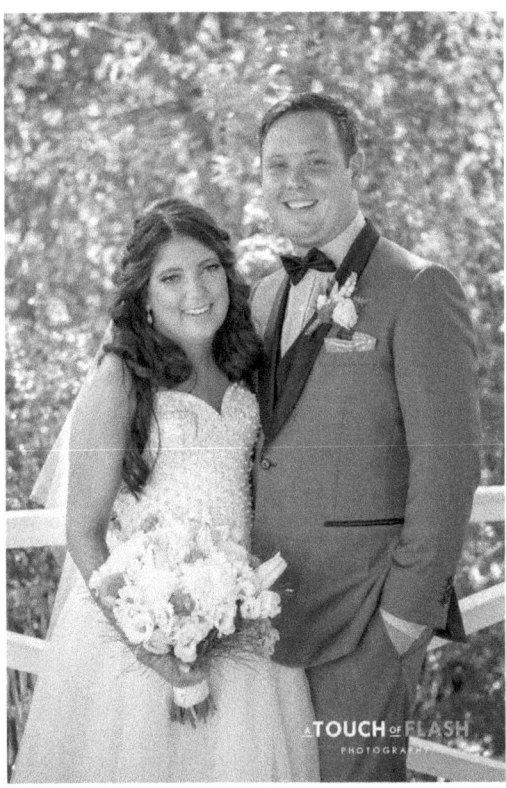

The next thing that was a high priority on my list was dance lessons. I always envisioned that my first dance with my husband was a beautiful choreographed dance. Something that was entertaining and different, similar to myself, nothing boring

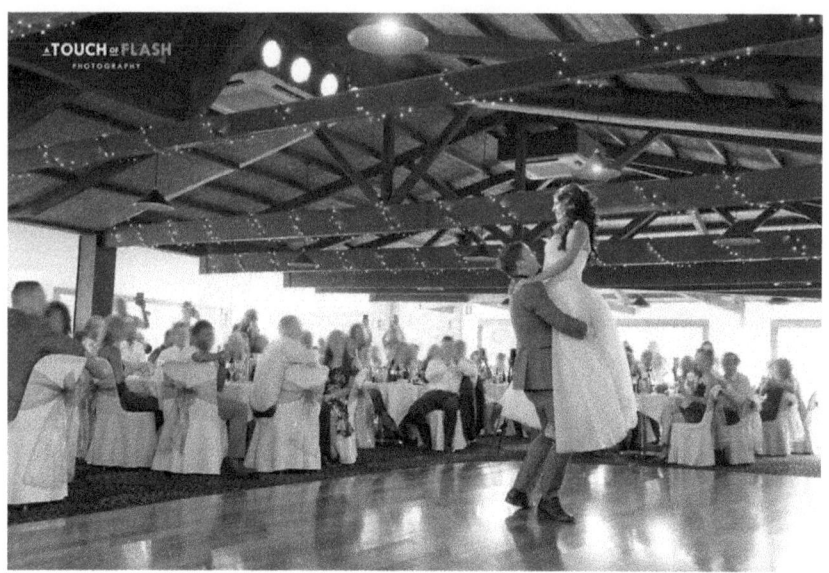

so we completed ten dance lesson leading up to the wedding on a Monday night and learnt and rehearsed what was to be our first dance. This is on my social media accounts if you want to have a look!

So you know that old tale of the bride always being late to her own wedding, like it was almost expected. Well, not in our case, Aaron was actually late to our wedding and I will tell you the reason why. We didn't need wedding cars to take us to our wedding because the venue had amazing facilities for us to get ready there, so therefore the room I was getting ready in lead straight to the isle of where the ceremony was hoping to be held. Aaron and his groom party decided to drive their beloved cars to the venue and display them. But there was one thing missing, and that was the ribbon that goes across the bonnet. Classic, disorganised Aaron thought it would be a good idea to stop at *Spotlight* on the way to get ribbon for the car but failed to leave that little bit of extra time. It didn't really matter though and became a story to tell about our day.

Our wedding was one of the best days of our lives, surrounded by family and friends, dancing all night, and just having pure fun. If something little didn't go to plan, we didn't care, we just brushed it off and continued to have a great night. The dreaded speeches, they are either entertaining or boring. They either go too long or too short. We limited everyone to two minutes each as we knew they had to be done but we were also so eager to continue the celebrations. It was Aarons turn to talk now and he was so nervous, again, he had not prepared anything so spoke from his heart. He got so emotional that he could not even finish his speech. An event would not be complete if Emmilia had not taken over in some way so that's what I did, grabbed the microphone and just started talking. I could not even tell you what I said as I made it up on the spot. I think I made everyone laugh so I was happy.

Remember earlier when I said that I would use any excuse for a party? Yeah, well, I had organised an after party at our house the very next day at 12pm. We woke up at 9am from our wedding, got home by 10am, my hair and makeup was still perfect, put a summer dress on and started making Bolognese sauce to serve as one of the dishes to the fifty guests that were coming over at 12pm. The kitchen was jam packed with helpers trying to set everything up and then the day was celebrated. There is no better feeling than creating simple and happy memories with people around you that matter the most.

To us, that is priceless.

CHAPTER 9

ALOHA BITCHES

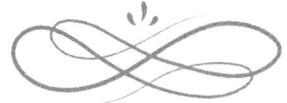

When Aaron and I visit a place, whether it is local in Victoria or another state of Australia, or even another country, we love to explore that place as much as we can to the point where we almost need another holiday to recover from our original holiday.

Where was our honeymoon going to be? The weather had to be warm and it had to be a place that had many things to do. A place we had never been to before but always wanted to visit one day and preferably overseas as who knows when the next opportunity was going to be for us to go overseas. Oh and the place had to have some sort of zoo/animal experience, that seemed to be our thing now as we love animals so much. We also had to choose a place that was going to be within our budget too. We had already been to Bali and Thailand before.

Sunny Queensland and Sydney were also places we had been too. Europe and Mainland USA were not an option as we only had ten days and not a huge budget so Hawaii was the option and we were so excited.

A couple of days after the wedding, we jumped onto our scheduled approx. direct thirteen hour Jetstar flight straight to Honolulu to spend the next ten days there. And I am not exaggerating when I say it was jam packed, we pretty much had something planned every day.

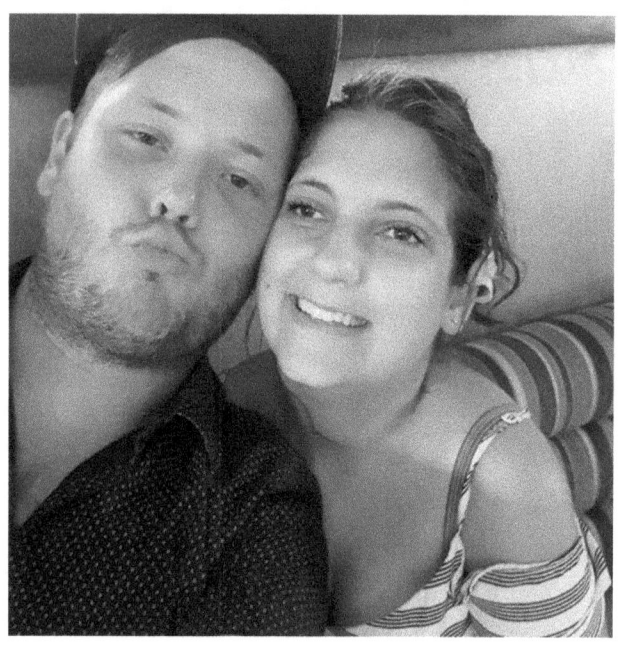

We spent three full days shopping at the outlets and the main shopping centre, we had to purchase a third suitcase so we were able to bring everything home! Some of the experiences we were lucky to be involved in was a helicopter ride to see the picturesque island and then the next day, the total opposite on the ocean floor in a submarine. A traditional luau dinner was so inviting as it was a Hawaiian feast with love, music and vibrant cultural performances. Speaking of dinners, another night we set sail on the water and enjoyed a sunset dinner cruise as a married couple. We took a mini flight to the Island of Hawaii for a day to go on a Volcano experience, the tour guide was amazing and we actually got to walk on top of an active volcano. Discovered that volcanic rock is very light and got to touch/carry it.

Also learnt that you still need your passport if you take a domestic flight in another country and not just your Driver's License from Australia. The amazing airport staff still let us on the plane, however we had to get frisked search on the way there and on the way back, I guess we can tick that off some sort of bucket list!

It didn't stop there; if you ever go to Hawaii, you MUST attend and spend the day at the Polynesian Cultural Centre. It was my favourite day of the holiday. Lastly, Pearl Harbor, I have always been interested in learning about this part of history and I was privileged enough to walk on the same grounds and take in the horrendous moment of history that happened on the 7th of December 1941. At Pearl Harbor, you get the privilege to witness the sunken ship that lies beneath the water, and the feeling of emotions when you are there is so overwhelming; the feeling is so hard to describe. You literally are taken to the site of the ship via a boat and stand directly on top of the sunken ship. You look down and see the ship right beneath you and instantly think of all of the buried souls that are stuck in the remains of the ship and never returned to their loved ones.

You suddenly forget everything else that is going on in the world and your life because they don't matter at this point in time as you start to feel grateful to be alive.

No matter what is going on in your life, treat each day like it is your last and live your life to the best of your ability.

I was stable again and got cleared from all of my doctors that I was healthy and results were coming back normal. The existing tumours were just there again so I continued my life.

Kidney was doing great again, the best function I had in a long time so it clearly just meant I needed to visit Hawaii more often.

Towards the end of 2018, my family and I decided it was time to embark on purchasing and running our own business. So we bought a family fish and chip shop. We thought it was perfect timing, my health was great so I could focus on a job. Mum was going to be out of her second job soon as that business was closing down. It seemed right.

Being part of a business owner is tough work, you literally are working twenty-four hours, seven days a week. Not only do you have to work in the business physically during opening hours, you also have to organise everything in the background too from ordering to bookwork and everything in between.

We all learnt new sides to each other, really tested our relationship and boundaries but there is one thing we can be proud of, and that was that we took a severely rundown business on the verge of closing down and flipped it over and made it great again.

A usual protocol for women receiving a kidney transplant or I would imagine any transplant is that you have to have a contraceptive plan in place for at least one to two years after surgery.

I chose to have the *Implanon* device, also known as 'the rod', inserted into my arm, it lasts three years and if it works for you, then you do not have to worry about it so that's what I did, in fact I had a total of two devices inserted back to back over six years. The plus side was that I didn't have to deal with the womanly monthly cycle either.

In December 2019 the device was due to be removed, my health was stable, the business was stable so again, perfect timing for Aaron and I to start looking into family planning and investigate starting a family. As my history was so complex, everything had to be looked into and approved before we could start so we knew it was going to be a long process.

Step one, the rod was removed and I had to wait for my menstrual cycle to begin again as that is essential in the baby making process. Then that dreading waiting process again, will I wake up today and receive my period? No. Three months had passed, three months of waiting and nothing so I brought this up with my doctor at the time. I was told to wait six months in total as sometimes things can take that little bit longer to kick start. Okay, so I continued to wait because we don't ever question the doctor, right?

During the grueling waiting time, Mum was due to turn fifty so what did we decide to do, surprise her with a ten day holiday to Hawaii. Aaron and I were off to Hawaii again to relive our honeymoon exactly two years later with my parents and younger brother. Hawaii was officially my happy place.

We were very fortunate and will be forever grateful to be able to go on this holiday as we had the business at the time and had no idea what was to come when we got back to the homeland,

Australia. We were in the lift at our resort in Hawaii and another guest from America was also in there too, and mentioned that someone at the resort had COVID-19. What the hell was COVID-19 and what did that mean? We researched a little bit on Google but did not learn much as it was so new back in February 2020. We just thought it was a flu-like cold and that we just had to be a little more careful around the resort. We were due to leave in a couple of days anyway so we did not think much of it.

Before we knew it, we were back at home, working in our business and living a normal life until we heard the word COVID-19 being talked about more and more often. Cases were soaring and life was put on hold with lockdowns. Hospitals were filling up quickly and businesses were closing down. People were losing their physical lives and livelihoods, it was scary.

I was so genuinely scared for humanity that I wrote a letter and plead to the premier Dan Andrews at the time to think about the everyday Australian and our medical system. I was worried for our medical system and how the staff were going to cope in a system that was already on the verge of falling apart. What about people like me who had chronic and deadly medical conditions, were there going to be beds available for us if we needed them? Staff to keep us alive? **I COULD HAVE F'N DIED!** I also felt for the people who had worked their whole lives and then had their business or home ripped apart from them almost overnight. How were people going to live and survive?

My letter ended up in the Leader Newspaper but that's about it, I never received a response.

As a result of my past medical history, not only do I live with cancer every single day, I also have other chronic conditions that I endure as a result like Osteoporosis which is a condition of the bones and their inability to regenerate quickly enough. Hypothyroidism (underactive thyroid) is an autoimmune disease.

Developing Osteoporosis in my twenties was confronting, I thought this was something that happened way later on in life when I got old. The amount of steroids I have consumed, and still continue to consume today, along with the kidney disease, has ruined my bone density. Although I have never broken a bone!

Exercise, if you do not like it like me, is hard. It is so hard to work up the motivation to even present to a gym, let alone actually participate if you are not a fan of exercise. This is where my good friend Linda steps in again and kept me accountable. There really is no treatment for Osteoporosis other than feeding calcium to the bones and exercise to keep them strong so I had to learn to enjoy it because I was and still am determined to never break a bone.

You would never know if you had Osteoporosis unless you encountered a bone fracture and had a bone densisty scan. It is a silent bone disease that consists of the body loosing bone and then not being able to make enough bone to replace the lost bone, resulting in a higher risk of fractures.

Hypothyroidism is just annoying, the symptoms are awful and include tiredness, feeling cold all of the time, weight gain to name a few. You have to consume daily tablets in the morning at the same time, half an hour before food and no dairy within two hours, who made up these rules? Attend regular blood tests and are forever adjusting the dose as the levels fluctuate so much. It's very high maintenance.

Let's go to June 2020 now, we are deep into the COVID-19 pandemic and family planning is still on the cards. Still had that one problem of no menstrual cycle so it was back to the doctors for step three; further tests to find out what was going on.

I was to undertake a full hormone panel blood test to see what the hormones were doing in my body. They all came back a flat out *zero*, nothing. I had none and nothing was happening. That explains the absent menstrual cycle. Next test was a MRI of the brain and head. MRI stands for Magnetic Resonance Imaging and uses magnets in a machine to take images. You have to be extremely still and not wear any metal.

There is a tiny little gland that lives below the brain around the middle of your head called the Pituitary Gland and this gland is predominantly responsible for regulating hormones and sending signals to the brain to order the body to do particular things. In a females case, tell the brain to remind the reproductive system to create and then release an egg every month and if that egg is not fertlised, get rid of it via a period. So I have the MRI and I get the results and they are not good.

There is no such thing has perfect timing, is it ever the right time to do anything? Never is.

CHAPTER 10

CRANIOTOMY 101

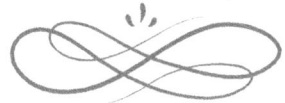

Results came in and a lesion was found in my pituitary gland region, and I had to undergo another biopsy. This time the biopsy was through my nose to verify what the lesion was.

I just knew at this stage it was going to be another smooth muscle tumour, because I mean, what else was it going to be? It was the same scenario, scan, lesion found, biopsy, smooth muscle tumour, some unknown treatment. They were literally going to stick something up my nose and enter my head cavity and take a piece of me. *I thought we were taught to never stick anything up our nose when we were young?*

I don't have to tell you, you already know, a smooth muscle tumour was confirmed in my head, and it was big, three to four centimetres. I would have never even known it was there if I wasn't family planning as I didn't have any other symptoms, and who knows how long it was there for *and* growing. It needed to come out, it was so close to the nerves around my right eye too that not only was it causing the menstrual issues, it was bound to affect my eyesight.

It all happened so quickly, within a week of the biopsy, I was in the doctor's office discussing the results and coming up with a plan. Initially I was told that they may be able to remove it from my nose. I imagined it was going to be like them removing a big booger while I was asleep but then it was discovered that it was too large and the best approach was a to remove it via my head.

A *Craniotomy* is a surgery to remove the skull to expose the brain and surrounding areas.

Hang on one second, surgery was scheduled in August 2020, deep in a medical world pandemic and my head was just about to be cut open and my brain exposed to remove an unwanted mass of cells…

Okay, let's just do it and get it over with.

The craniotomy may not have been enough to remove the whole tumour so I was also warned that I may have to be in hospital for an extra week and complete a second surgery, transsphenoidal removal. These surgeries are performed by Neurosurgeons and Ear Nose Throat (ENT) Surgeons.

I knew I was going to be in hospital for at least one week but may have possibly been two weeks, and I was strictly not allowed to have any visitors the whole entire time. This was the hardest part to understand and was going to be the hardest part to deal with as in the past I always had a visitor to keep my spirits high and keep me motivated. I understood the reasoning behind it though, and that reasoning was that it was to ensure I stayed safe as I absolutely could *not* contract COVID-19 during this time, but I had never felt so alone in my life.

My husband drove me to the hospital early the morning of my head surgery. I had to be there at 7am, and it felt like I was being abandoned although I knew the place I was being dropped off to so well. The feeling of knowing that I was going to spend at least one week at a place I knew so well but hated so much with no familiar people around me did not sit with me well at all.

It all happened so quickly: I presented at the admissions department, went through all the usual ID checks and medical questions. Changed into the embarrassing surgery gown, and within one hour of arriving at the hospital the anesthetist was ready for me and I was wheeled off to theatre to face the most invasive and scary surgery of my life. I wasn't scared of the actual surgery or the fact that my head was about to be cut open, I was scared of the aftermath, the recovery. Was I going to lose my eyesight, have brain damage? Was the tumour even going to be able to be removed? Was I just about to participate in a life threatening surgery all for nothing? **I COULD END UP F'N DEAD!**

Now I am in the pre theatre room, again, I have been in this room countless of times, I know exactly what is coming and my anxiety kicks in. Happens every damn time. No one around me knows this but literally five minutes before every surgery or anesthetic experience, I start to cry uncontrollably, my body starts shaking and I am genuinely scared. I just want to get up and run. A sense of pain comes over me and I suddenly start to remember all of the horrible medical experiences I have endured. I can't control the feeling and start saying to the medical staff that I feel silly for feeling this way and I don't know what is wrong with me. I think I am having an anxiety attack. Every time without fail, the beautiful medical staff reassure me and tell me that I am doing so well. Certainly does not feel like it, I feel weak and useless, a burden!

It never made any sense to me because I know that I would and will be okay. Then I realised, it was all about losing the sense of control. As soon as the medication hits your vein, you are out within seconds and you are unable to control that feeling. No matter what you do, you are destined to fall asleep and not wake up until the doctors allow it.

First the calming medication is injected and suddenly I feel happy and I am smiling and laughing, talk about from one extreme to another. I start to become annoying as now I am just a chatterbox and annoying to the medical staff. Then the next dose goes in and I am out.

Many hours later, I wake up and I am in recovery, pretty sure the surgery was all day. I am so confused and so drowsy. So many tubes coming out of me everywhere, staples across my head and covered with a white bandage. My right eye is swollen, shut and bruised. The vision in my left eye a little blurry but I am pain free. It seriously looked like I had entered the biggest boxing match ever and got destroyed.

It's the next day and the morning nurse happily greet me and then tell me I need to sit up and take a few steps. How was I supposed to do this, my balance is terrible, tubes and cords everywhere, I can barely see but I did it. One step at a time.

There was a process because all of my facial muscles were weak as they took a hit, my right eye was closed and my left eye lid did not have the strength to stay open so I improvised. I literally taped my left eyelid open so I could at least see. The font on my phone was so big that you could see it from a mile away and I was on so much pain relief medication that I could not hold anything properly. I also had a screw in my skull now to hold the bone together so now I can safely say that I do not have any screws loose!

I use the electric bed to sit up, I know, cheated a little but then I slowly proceeded to swing one leg over the side of the bed, with the nurses help of course. This alone took around half an hour. My head wanted to just get up and start walking but my body refused. I was handed a walking frame and now had to try and stand up, I had no strength at all. This was going to be near impossible.

In my head, I count one two three and try to stand up, nothing. I try again and nothing again. Now it becomes frustrating because two days ago, I could easily do this. Something as simple as standing up was the most difficult task for me at this point. With a little push from the nurse, I was finally up on my feet, success! It felt great but then I had to try and take a step. It was hard, and the smallest step I had ever taken I reckon; it was barely a step, but I did it. It took everything out of me and I had huge assistance but I still did it, it was a little win and I took it.

I spent most of the rest of the week sleeping, eating the blandest food ever, talking on the phone with my parents and husband and going for very short walks. It was so repetitive and driving me crazy. I could not watch much on my phone as light sensitivity was a real issue and then I would just fall asleep. I was trapped in a white room with white walls and a white floor dressed in a white gown covered with white bandages. I hate the colour white.

Just when I thought I was due to go home; I got the news that I had been dreading. We have to complete the *Transsphenoidal Surgery* to remove one-hundred-percent of the tumour. This meant another major surgery, another week in hospital and more time without seeing my family.

Naturally you would think that getting your head cut open would be worse than going through your nose but I was wrong. Two words; *skin graft*. Not only were they going to remove the rest of the tumour via my nose, they also had to grab some skin from the side of my thigh and reconstruct the internal nose and head cavity.

You know the drill now, theatre, anesthetic, operation, recovery room, back to the ward and recovery. This was slightly different, woke up in recovery and was faced with unexpected excruciating pain that was coming from my thigh. So painful that I think I screamed the hospital down. So many medical staff trying to assist and work out what was the issue. I did not know at the time that the skin graft was causing the pain either. Of course, after a lot of pain relief, I was somewhat comfortable.

It was now my second week in hospital and it was the same thing on repeat but now my biggest concern was my right eye and eye lid. The eye lid was shut and purple. No feeling in or around it, I could not even move my eye brow. Everything was stiff and all I got told was to wait as it could take up to twelve weeks to recover and open. *Twelve weeks! Three months!* I wanted it open now because my plans were to go home and resume my normal life as quickly as possible. Surgeries were done and I was ready to forgot about them and move on now.

Staple removal day, the thick twenty plus staples that ran across the front and side of my head were going to be picked out one by one. First the bandage comes off and I can tell you now, the worst part of anything medical is ripping a sticky bandage off. It hurts and all of your fine little hairs are ripped out. I don't use waxing services and this is why! Then the nurse picks up some sort of tool and starts to remove the staples. I am terrified, the noise and then feeling of them coming out was unlike anything I had ever felt before. What was five minutes felt like five hours and then they were out and it was like it was nothing. I was freaking myself out for nothing!

I am finally given the all clear to go home and I am well, at this stage I could complete two to three full laps around the ward of walking, which killed some time every day. I ring Aaron straight away and tell him to pick me up in the morning. I am so excited I get to leave the prison of the hospital and go to familiar territory, eat a delicious home cooked meal, and be surrounded by my family.

When I got home, I quickly learnt that my recovery was going to be long and grueling. It was not going to be as simple as waking up and going about my normal day. I had to deal with having one eye lid shut, the daily pain and knowing that I needed help with any task I was to complete whether that was big or small. We also had to arrange for someone to be with me at all times as the risk of seizure was so high in the first three months. I was not allowed to drive for three months post-surgery in case I was to have a seizure and if I did, those three months would have to start again. I had a rotating roster between my parents, Aaron's mum, and Aaron. I do not know what I would have done if I had no one in my life.

I was unable to make any meals or even get up on my own. I was unable to watch something for long or have bright light around me. I lost all independence and any ability to do the simple things in life like reading, walking, and *seeing*. I also lost the things I loved doing the most: driving and cooking. I felt useless.

Weeks went by and I attended all of my hospital appointments and check-ups. My right eye lid had no bruising anymore but I was still unable to open it. I started doing eye brow exercises to get that moving again too. I kept being told to wait and I started to question it; we were two months post surgery and there was no sign of my right eye lid opening, not even a little. Aaron and I decided to read my twenty-page long discharge summary again to see if we could find some sort of note in there in regards to my eye lid and then we read, "Third Fourth Cranial Nerve Sacrificed."

My heart sank; the nerve that controls the eye lid from moving up and down was sacrificed, severed, cut, broken and not coming back.

Not one medical staff member mentioned about my nerve being sacrificed and Aaron and I questioned this to various medical staff members at the hospital after reading the discharge summary again including the Neuro Surgeon, ENT Surgeon and Opthamologist.

We never got a proper answer out of them, we were told that we just had to wait or it appears that it will be permanently shut.

I was devastated knowing that I was going to look like this forever, we even investigated the possibility of another surgery to lift the eye lid but because the eye ball also does not move and has lost all feeling, the risk of dry eye and infections are way too high. Initially, I wore a white medical bandage eye patch and pretended that I had eye surgery but I couldn't do this forever. I tried to tape it and glue it open for events but that just hurt. I developed a new hair style that would have a fringe come across half of my face to hide the eye.

My confidence was shot and not coming back anytime soon. I enter a shopping centre or a place and people stare. I know they don't mean it and they are just curious but you can feel them starring straight at you. I meet new people and cannot look them in the eye for fear of them staring back at me in disgust. I am afraid to go out in public with family and friends as I am scared for them and their embarrassment of being around me, a person with one eye. I can't look in the mirror and be happy with myself and the way I look. How was I ever going to meet new people confidently and obtain a job. Children and Kids would be scared to look at me. When people look at me, what do they think of me? When I am with my husband or parents, do people automatically think I have a carer? I have tried to live my life so independently and now I would have to rely on everyone for everything. What about my husband? He did not marry someone with one eye. What was he going to think of me every time he looked at me? I felt I was no longer attractive. The constant questions from everyone was 'When is your eye going to open?' or 'You will be better when you get your eye opened up' or 'You will feel normal again one day.' This whole time I knew that it was never going to open up.

What is *normal*? Something standard, typical, usual and expected.

There is no normal; everyone has a different 'normal'. What is usual for one may be unusual for another. That is the beauty of life; everyone is unique in their own way that we can learn so much from others.

What makes it so much worse is that I usually do not care what people think of me but I kept letting this get to me and I did not like it so my attitude towards it had to change and it did.

Yes, I wear my hair a certain way and yes I still do not like looking at myself in a mirror but I remind myself every day of what I have been through and I am still here and survived.

Let people stare if they want too and shut down the unwanted thoughts that run through my mind. At the end of the day, this is me now and I have to accept it and I did. I meet new people all the time now and go out with family and friends constantly. I complete a visual field study eye test every two years and I am able to drive again. I have learnt to live with my new appearance because appearance does not change your personality and beliefs. I am still the same person on the inside, I just look a little different. At least I can say that I am a one eyed Collingwood supporter now.

One-hundred-percent of the tumour was removed and I was alive so I will take that as a win and am so thankful.

CRANIOTOMY 101

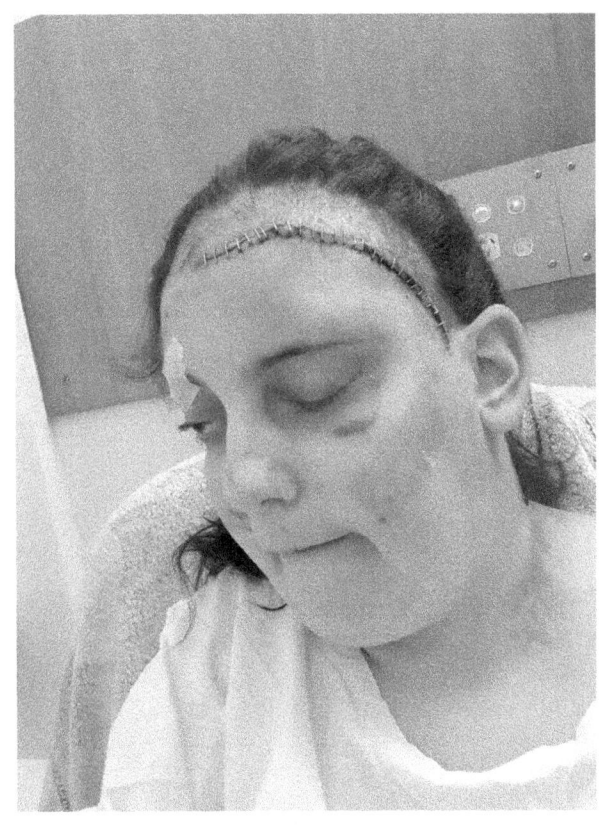

CHAPTER 11

THE DECISIONS OF INCISIONS

Three months after my head surgery, November 2020 (notice I don't call it brain surgery, I find that head surgery sounds nicer), I attended my routine post surgery appointment with the ENT surgeon to check progress.

At this stage, I was pretty much back to my usual self, I was driving, cooking and living. I was lined up to start my personal training sessions again and just had to work out what type of job I was going to apply for because I was so bored at home every single day, doing the same thing over and over again.

I asked the surgeon out of curiosity if the tumours on both sides of my neck could ever be removed in the future as they were getting quite large and painful to lay on. I was not in a rush and I just wanted to know if it was ever going to be a possibility.

The surgeon did not object to it but of course an MRI was ordered to check the structure and confirm if it was a possibility, and a follow up appointment was made in a couple of months.

Within a week of completing the MRI, I received a phone call and was asked to attend an appointment in a couple of days to receive the results. I was confused and knew something bad was coming. I must have to remove these neck tumours sooner rather that later were my initial thoughts.

I nervously attend my appointment alone because I had a feeling that I was not going to get great news and everytime I had brought a family member with me, they would start crying, and I did not want to have to deal with that again! People may think this is strange as people usually bring a family or friend to support them in a tough situation but let's not forget that I was usually the support person to others in my tough situation.

The surgeon called me in and starts to ask me if I have any pain in my neck. I responded the usual symptom of the side of my neck hurt when I am lying down on one of the tumours but that's about it.

The surgeon then says, "What about the back of the neck? The Spine?"

I respond, "No."

"Well Emmilia, your c5 vertebrae is fractured."

I look at the surgeon and ask, "How?" I hadn't done any dare devil activities, nor had I had a fall.

"You have a tumour in the vertebrae, and because your bones are so fragile it has fractured it."

My world came crashing down, I had just finally somewhat recovered from my last two serious surgeries and now I was going to be up for another one. This was going to be worse than the two before as they were going to be working on my spine. The good news was that they could remove the tumours on the sides of my neck at least.

Remember always see the good things in any situation right?

The surgery was going to involve a neck dissection on both sides of my neck, removing the tumour in my spine via the front of my neck and then inserting a cage through the front of my neck to hold the vertebrae in place. So basically two surgeries at once.

A neck dissection is a surgery to removes tissues or tumours in the neck, this can include lymphnodes. Anterior Lumbar Interbody Fusion (ALIF) which is a procedure used to stabilize the spine and gains access through the front of the neck.

Surgery was booked in for Tuesday the 29th of December 2020. I was allowed to celebrate Christmas but knew I was going to be in hospital for New Year's Eve, but it didn't really worry me like usual. I thought, *let's just hurry up and have the surgery so I can start to recover and move on with my life.* This is my thought pattern every time I am presented with a medical diagnosis.

It was the usual scenario again but this time I woke up in the Intensive Care Unit (ICU) with about twenty staples on both sides of my neck, and wearing a neck brace. I did not know if the surgery went well at this stage but I was guessing not as planned since I was in ICU. I was stable but I needed to be watched every minute as I was unable to move. It was too dangerous; I could run the risk of damaging my spinal cord and therefore not being able to walk again. This actually scared me and I like to think that not much in the medical world scares me.

My only thoughts were, *do anything and everything I can to avoid that situation and stay as still as possible. Don't move.* I was on so many pain relievers that I slept most of the time anyway.

I woke up the next morning and was greeted by the surgeon who said the neck dissections went really well and the tumour in the vertebrae was removed however my bones were not great at all and they were worried that the c5 vertebrae was unlikely to recover. I had two options:

Option one was to stay in a neck brace for six weeks and then have a scan to see if the bone was recovering, and if the bone was not recovered I would need to have a spinal fusion. And option two was to forget about the six week wait and go straight into surgery tomorrow and complete a spinal fusion to secure everything and get rid of the neck brace straight away.

It was actually an easy decision, why wait on the small chance that I would not require the surgery to probably find out that I would need it all along anyway?

Recover from my current neck dissections to then go back to square one with another surgery and start the recovery process again. Option two, surgery, it was!

I just wanted to start recovering again so I could continue my life. So it was New Year's Eve and I went into surgery again for the surgeons to perform a spinal fusion in which they had to connect multiple bones from the spine. The fusion would be eight levels, from c2 to t1, which is massive. Two rods side by side would be installed and plenty of screws to hold it all together.

I don't wake up from the fusion surgery, I am put into an induced coma as my neck started to swell as I could not breathe properly.

I missed New Year's Eve and most of the morning of the first day in 2021. **HOW AM I NOT F'N DEAD!**

> *"I know you cant read this right now but I just want to say I love you so much! I'm so sorry that you have had to be kept asleep for New Years and you dont even know it right now. I'm sorry that I didn't talk to you before your surgery and tell you how much I love you.*
>
> *I missed you so much tonight, you are the best thing that ever happened to me and I can't live without you. Happy New Year even though you have missed it and hopefully 2021 will be a better year for you and us! — feeling heartbroken."* – Aaron O'Sullivan (Facebook Post on the 1st of January 2021)

At this time, the COVID-19 pandemic started to slightly get better and I was allowed two visitors for two hours a day. I wake up and see my parents smiling back at me but I am unable to speak as I have a tube down my throat. People that know me know that I love to talk, so not being able to talk was very unusual and confronting. My little mind ticked and I started drawing letters on the blanket with my finger and the nurse instantly knew that I wanted to say something so she grabbed a small white board and a marker for me.

I simply wrote, "When will this tube come out?"

Everyone started laughing and the nurse said very soon, and very soon after the tube was pulled out and I could speak again but barely. Due to the surgery being near my vocal cords and throat muscles, I initially lost my voice and ability to swallow water and food. The muscles were compromised so I had to result in a feeding tube for nutrients and fluids through the drip for water. Talking was more of a whisper and it hurt but it never stopped me. I just had to talk slower and softly for a while. In hindsight, I probably should have learnt to be quiet so I could recover quicker.

A couple of days later and I was back on the general ward to start my whole recovery process again. The usual getting up and walking everyday, but this time it was so much harder. Just imagine twenty staples on each side of your neck and a neck brace tightly around the neck pushing on those staples. No muscles left anywhere around your body and unable to lift your left hand passed your shoulder. Yep, that was me. The pain was real; one ever so slight movement and it felt like agony. A persons mind has such great power and mine was constantly telling me to just 'Hurry up, get up and start walking' but my physical body was unable to do this. I just wanted it all to be over and I wanted to go back in time when I was stable and living my life but I knew the next six months were going to be grueling and that I had to focus on the little wins as that was what was going to get me to my end long term goal.

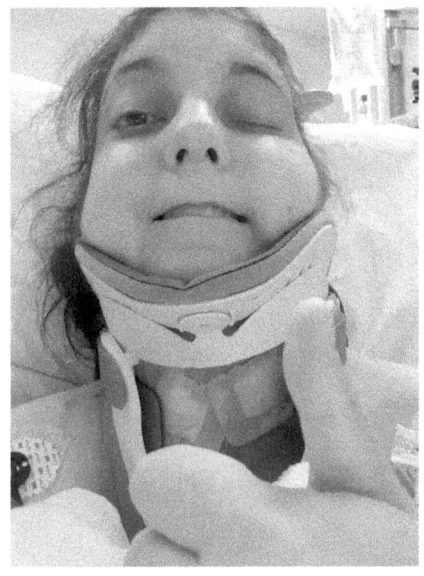

Before I could even think about working on my physical strength, I had to sort out the eating and drinking situation. First was trying to consume water, I could not take a sip without it going down the wrong way and choking. I tried small sips, larger sips, using a straw and I even used a syringe at one point to control how much liquid I would have. I started sucking on ice to stay hydrated, but nothing was working.

For someone who only drinks water and a minimum of two litres per day, this was a serious problem. I am known to be a water connoisseur; I *can* taste good water from bad water. Yes, it has

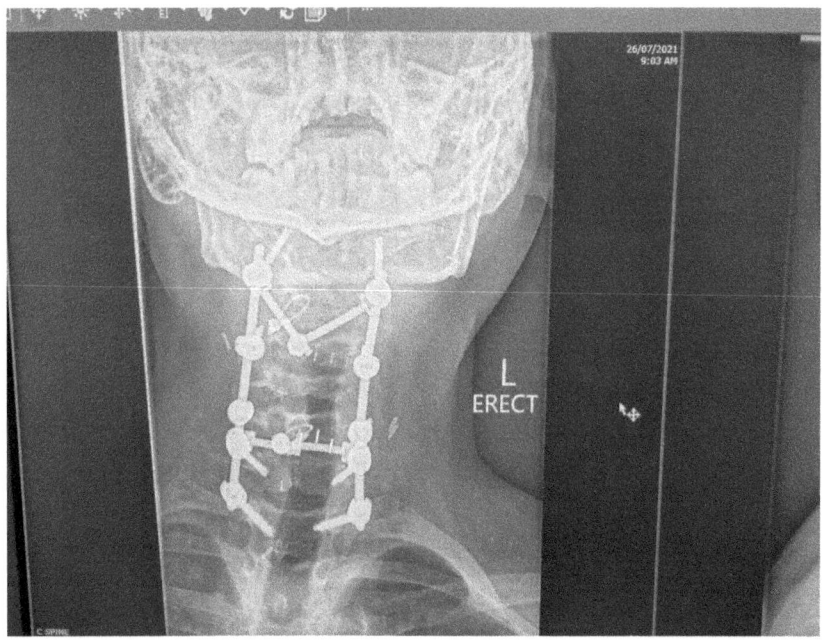

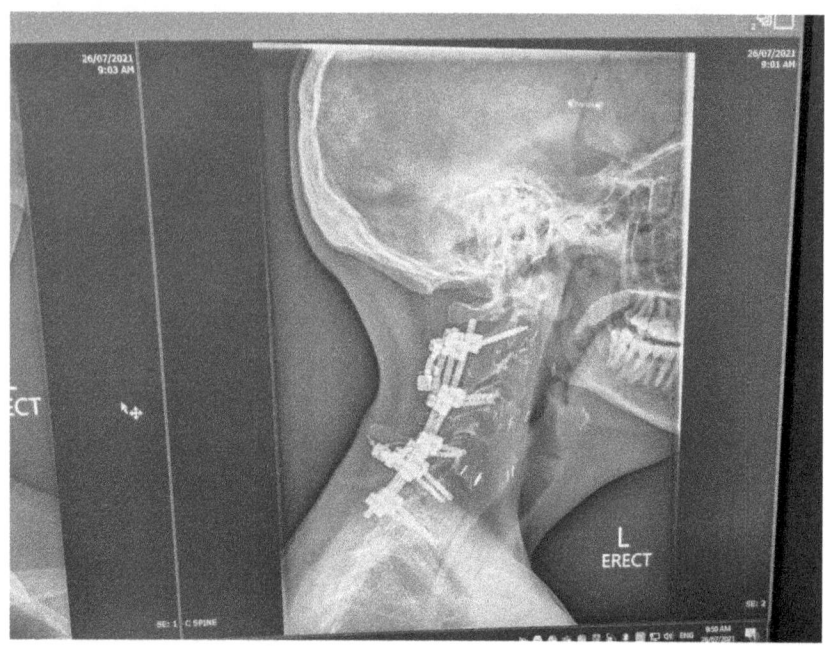

a taste. We have a 'magic' fridge at home, one of those side by side fridges that has the water filter and ice maker, I often can tell when the water starts to not taste right and report to Aaron that the filter will need to be changed soon and almost every time within one week of making the declaration, the change filter light turns on.

The dietician payed me a visit on the ward and introduced me to an agent that I had to put in anything liquid to thicken it up. Except, it had to be the correct consistency, not too thick or thin or I would choke, it had to be just right! Even just right was not so right, it was horrible, tasted like water but weird, the texture was all so wrong, when I got home, I landed myself back in hospital for a few days to get hydrated again.

The dietician was also concerned about my nutrition and how I was going to get nutrition into my body. I didn't need the feeding tube anymore because I could somewhat handle thickened soup and mash potato and gravy. Soups and mash along with some Sustagen Nutritional Drink and I pretty much lived on that the whole time I was in hospital. I was offered pureed mince meat and declined it very quickly. The texture and smell was so wrong, like dog food. When I got home, I had to create a baby food diet full of puree food. Food consisted of pureed pumpkin soup, mash potato and gravy, pureed broccoli and cauliflower just to name a few.

There is nothing worse than sitting around a table with everyone who can eat all of the foods and you are stuck with a bland puree.

This went on for two whole months until I could tolerate some sort of solid food and when I could tolerate solid food, I would need to chew and chew and chew before I even thought of swallowing it. I was already an extremely slow eater so this experience just took slow eating to a whole new level. I would be served my food before anyone else's food was even cooked and I would still be trying to eat by the time they had cooked and eaten their food.

The car ride home was not fun at all. Neck brace was on along with the staples, then partnered with every single little bump was destined to hurt so much and it did. Over the course of being home for a week, I complained every day that something was digging into my neck and no amount of pain relief was giving me the relief I needed. At discharge, I was told that I had to wear the brace for two weeks at home until my follow up appointment but then I remember being told that if I was to have the fusion, I shouldn't need the neck brace. I was so confused as to why I had the neck brace on, so due to barely having a voice, Mum gets on the phone to the surgeon.

The surgeon apologised and gave me the all clear to remove the neck brace over the phone and suddenly I was scared. I immediately thought that as soon as I removed the brace, my neck would not be able to support itself and flop to one side. I can confirm, this did not happen and laugh about it now.

I was now settled nicely in my home, I had aids like a shower chair and bed rail to try and make simple tasks a little easier. I was unable to wash my hair because I couldn't lift my arm but I persevered. The rotating roster came back in and I had different people come over every day to keep me company and make sure I was okay, but I needed to start my rehabilitation, build my strength again and become my independent self again. I hated relying on people and hated that I couldn't simply jump into my car and drive to the supermarket to get ingredients to then make dinner.

The hospital enrolled me in their six week rehabilitation program; this would have been around March 2021. A tailored program was made specifically for me after I initially performed some basic physical tests to determine my level of strength.

The program consisted of one on one training with the physiotherapist and then a one on one session with the exercise physiotherapist in the gym. I graduated the program and made huge progress, so now it was back to my friend Linda at Infinity 360. I got dropped off and picked up from the gym three times a week, and each week I made a little more progress. I started off completing a very slow and light movement workout. I honestly felt quite useless and embarrassed. Over the weeks, I started to see progress and the reality of recovering and being independent again suddenly becomes real. Soon enough, I was able to drive short distances and complete very light duties at home like washing a plate and filling up my water bottle.

THE DECISIONS OF INCISIONS

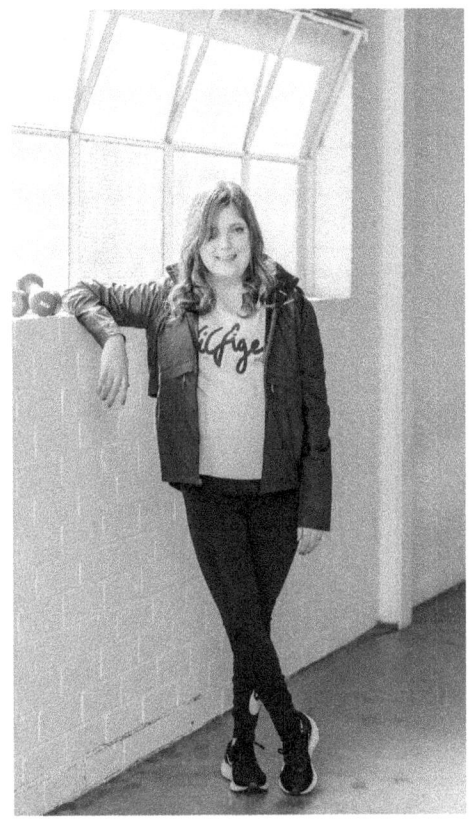

Baby steps, remember?

It would have been the middle of 2021 now and I wanted to enter back into the workforce because I was so bored at home but I had to work out what I could apply for. I always said to myself that it would be perfect if I could have a job working from home and work as required depending on how I felt and what appointments I had for the week. My medical issues were a part time job in itself, so much coordinating and having to be organised with appointments and ensure my supply of daily medication never ran out. Then having to make sure I stayed healthy by consuming good food and regularly exercising so I knew I was only dreaming when it came to finding the perfect stay at home job for me.

One day in June, I was scrolling through Facebook and found a local admin job on the suburb community page that was a work from home role. I instantly thought it was too good to be true, but I still applied as I had nothing to lose. Weeks passed and I heard nothing back, so I knew it was too good to be true!

Suddenly, out of nowhere, I get a call and was offered a phone interview the next day regarding job I had applied for weeks ago. I was so excited but nervous and now I didn't know what to say during the phone conversation. Do I tell them the truth? Do I pretend that there is nothing wrong with me? I decide to mention that I have some health conditions, however they are completely managed and that I did not care how many hours I worked. I just needed someone to give me the opportunity. That phone call landed me a zoom video interview and within a week I had started my new job as an admin assistant at Landmark Inspections.

This gave me a whole new purpose to life and gave me a reason to live and do it well. I was and still am dedicated to my job and can honestly say that I actually love my job. I run a department within the company now and treat it like I own it and will be forever grateful for my boss and manager for believing in me and giving me that one opportunity I needed.

They say 'good things come to those who wait'? Well, with a little patience and some effort, a good thing came to me.

CHAPTER 12

LIKE A PHOENIX, I RISE

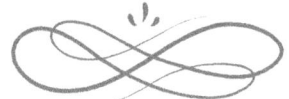

This brings us to the start of 2022, nearly there! Life was great again; I was managing my health superbly and working full time. I was getting stronger with my gym work and personal trainer.

All of these past years Aaron had supported me financially, physically and mentally. I strongly believe in the sayings, 'What goes around comes around' and, 'The tables turn around'. So, it was now my turn to return the favour.

An opportunity was presented to us and Aaron was given the option to start his own mechanical business, something that had always been the goal but was never the right time. *When is the right time again? Never.* Anyway, I gave him a little nudge as he was so apprehensive at the time and next thing we knew, we were in full swing of setting up his very own workshop from scratch. It was exciting and scary at the same time. If we succeeded, it would be great, if it went bust then we were at risk of losing our house, something that we had worked so hard to create and keep the past seven years. Aaron fully runs and operates the workshop all on his own to this day and he called it Fine Fix Mechanical. I was and am so proud of him for taking the step.

In October I was going to say goodbye to my twenties and join the thirties club and I was so eager to let them go. Most of my twenties was spent in hospitals completing surgeries; I needed a new beginning and was so determined to start my first year of turning thirty with a bang. It just was not the right bang I was looking for.

Of course, I had planned my party within three weeks, an abundance of food and dessert. Drinks galore with a person making yummy cocktails all night. Entertainment in the form of Drag Queens, that was fun. So much dancing with family and friends. Simply having a good time and making memories. It was perfect in my eyes or should I say eye.

Remember the last line from the first chapter, here it is again:

"Then the next thing I know I was on the stretcher and being wheeled out of my house and into the back of an ambulance on my way to the nearest Hospital Emergency Department."

I don't remember much of the Emergency Department that day of Sunday the 20th of November 2022 other than being wheeled into a resuscitation room and then darkness.

Not knowing that it was Sunday the 27th of November 2022 when I finally wake up and am conscious. I look around and realise I am in an ICU of a hospital, my second home at this stage. Initially I just think that I had a sleep and I have now awoken from it and had to come to ICU for a bad infection until I felt a tube down my throat again. I quickly realised I may have been asleep for a little longer than a couple of hours. The cause; sepsis. My instinct is to reach for the tube and pull it out myself and I am quickly stopped by the nurse and end up being shackled to the bed. I spend the next half an hour trying to wiggle my hands and wrists to break free from the bands, I had no hope but I was still going to try! A full week, seven days in an induced coma, I just lost one whole week of my life but that was not even the worst part.

This was the week from hell for everyone that knew me and I just slept peacefully throughout it all. Aaron, my parents, my brother and his girlfriend, my in-laws, brother-in-law, and sister-in-law, family and friends were told multiple times over the week that I would not make it and to prepare to say goodbye. My brother-in-law, who was overseas at the time, cut his trip short and flew back. I felt a little guilty about it, but it is nice to know that I do matter to people.

My organs were shutting down and I was on a life support machine to keep me alive.

To make things worse, two days into the coma, I suffered a cardiac arrest due to my blood pressure dropping so low and essentially died. CPR was needed to bring my back to life. **I WAS NEARLY F'N DEAD!**

Meeting after meeting with my parents, Aaron and the medical staff to report that I was not doing too well and that if I did even survive, there would not be much hope as my organs were no good. Brain damage was a real possibility and they could not even confirm that when the life machine would be turned off and the breathing tube come out of my mouth that I would even be able to breathe on my own anyway.

I can't even start to imagine how people would feel after witnessing and hearing this news, seeing a loved one in a hospital bed hooked up to so many machines and tubes. Unresponsive. Feeling helpless and praying that they are going to be okay, I am one of the lucky ones.

To be lucky is to receive something good, other words that you could use are fortunate or blessed but it's ironic. I consider myself lucky to be alive and to have survived what I have. Except none of it was good, and lucky can mean something completely different for someone else.

It was time to pull the breathing tube out and I was fully aware of what was about to happen and what could possibly happen.

This could be it and the last time I get to see my husband, he was the only one with me at the time, I stare at him and squeeze his hand so hard and the tube comes out and is immediately replaced with oxygen. *Obviously* I survive and take a breath but it is huge struggle. I wasn't going anywhere. I have so many more things to achieve in my life, I am not ready to leave. I have a fear of breathing masks so was not happy that I had to wear one but I knew it was the only thing that was helping me breath so I had no choice.

One of the first things I said to Aaron when the tube came out was, "Did you pay the gas bill?"

That was my number one priority the whole time I was asleep, the gas bill! I can confirm that the gas bill was paid and Aaron even made all of the other household required payments as he knew how organised I was with it all. Even though it took a phone call to the bank from him as he didn't know the repayment for our home loan and when I paid it. I promise our communication skills are getting better!

Next thing I wanted to do was sit up, I mean I had just spent the last week lying down so it was very reasonable. The bed transformed into a chair and I was alert and looking around surrounded by my family. Again, I was only allowed two visitors in my room at the time so it was another rotational roster between loved ones.

I was moved from my bed chair to a general chair and it felt so good to just sit up and be alive and breathe. Me being me, I was so eager to get up and walk but I did not have any shoes or footwear. My beautiful husband drove home and brought me back some slippers and safe to say I took a total of three steps and I was exhausted and done. Pretty sure I was running on adrenaline and the thrill of being alive.

My organs were working except my kidney, it had shut down and was not recovering. The doctors at the hospital told me that during my coma I was having dialysis and they advised that I needed to start again straight away but I was not convinced. I was scheduled to get a permacath inserted into my chest three days in a row so dialysis could commence but I refused it. I remembered back to the time when my native kidney failed and the creatinine test result came back in the 500's and was told that the kidney was failed and I required dialysis.

The doctors at the hospital were not my usual medical team, they did not know me or my history, and I was so complex that I had a gut feeling that they were wrong. My creatinine result while I was in hospital was around the 200 mark give or take, the doctors told me this was due to the dialysis I already had, but in my mind my kidney was not failing.

Yes, it was struggling but it was not failing.

Once you go on long term dialysis, there is no turning back and I was not prepared to lose this kidney, my gift of life. The little bean that was allowing me to live my life the way I was. This kidney still has so much to accomplish and it was not going anywhere.

I am on the ward now and I get worse, I lose all of my strength again, worst I have ever experienced ever. I could not hold my phone and a glass of water was too heavy. I could not sit up and was bedridden. The pain in my chest from the CPR is excruciating, I am pretty sure I have some sort of hairline fracture in the bones of my chest, a slight inhale was tormenting. All this time I had taken my strength and simple things in life for granted. It took all of these traumatic experiences to learn that walking and holding things are so simple and everyday functions for most people but can be taken away from you so quickly. Things that come so naturally to most now feel so unnatural.

Sitting in a hospital bed feeling helpless did not sit right with me so I begin my own plan for recovery. I ask the medical staff if I can see a physio to get me out of bed, they agree.

Over a couple of days, I learnt to walk again and sit in a chair next to my bed for most of the day. I was unable to get from my bed to the chair, or get up and start walking without assistance, but I felt like I somewhat accomplished something by sitting in a chair. When I sit in the chair, my laptop turns on and I start working on my work emails. I have literally come from my death bed and my priority now is to work and do my job.

Being in a coma for a whole week feels like the body has deteriorated to the point you have to start all over again by learning again. I got home and needed round the clock care, I could not even stand up from the couch and I was bound to a walking device. An old person's body was stuck with a young person's mind. I consulted Linda and we were video calling each other daily and completing exercises in the chair to try and get my blood moving and start to build my strength.

My whole world was flipped around and all I was focused on was making mine and Aaron's small trip to Canberra on the 2nd of January 2023 to visit Jamala Wildlife Park. I had waited a whole year for this trip and I was determined more than ever to show up and make it.

Jamala Wildlife Park is a zoo that has overnight accommodation directly with an animal, we chose the lion. In the room, a single piece of glass separating us and two lions all night. A lion would have to be my favourite animal as they are powerful, fierce and brave but so loyal.

We were due to spend four days in Canberra visiting the War Memorial, observing the Royal Australian Mint, and witnessing Parliament but the best place was saved for last, sleeping a night with real lions.

After spending three days at home being totally dependent on everyone around me, I visited my GP for a referral to any physical rehabilitation centre that would take me on two weeks before Christmas and I succeeded. Just after spending nearly three weeks in a hospital, I was now going to be admitted in the Donvale Rehab Facility to build my strength and fast. My goal was to at least be able to just get up and walk so I could go on the mini holiday.

The next ten days were spent completing four separate exercise sessions per day, it was intense and it was hard. Day one, I could not get up without assistance and could barely pick up a glass of water. I enter the group sessions and I am surrounded by people who are more than double my age. Each day things became easier, by day four or five, I ditched the walking frame and was becoming steadier on my feet. I was able to pour myself a glass of water.

Within ten days, I had made a 50% improvement and was released back to home on Christmas Eve just in time to celebrate Christmas. I also made it to my mini holiday in Canberra.

The first half of this year, 2023, I have really focused on building my strength. I ensure strength training is part of my routine, three times a week at minimum. I have learnt that the human body is so precious and it has to be looked after. The body is a vessel that allows us to complete simple and complex things but can be so easily damaged.

Do not get me wrong, I am so guilty of consuming pleasurable food and having a sneaky alcoholic drink from time to time but I am also the strongest I have ever physically been.

Every day is a struggle but only if I allow it to be but I can state today that I am a survivor and I have fought so hard to be here to tell the tale.

I should be F'N Dead! But I am not and the next mission in life is to create life so that brings us to IVF…

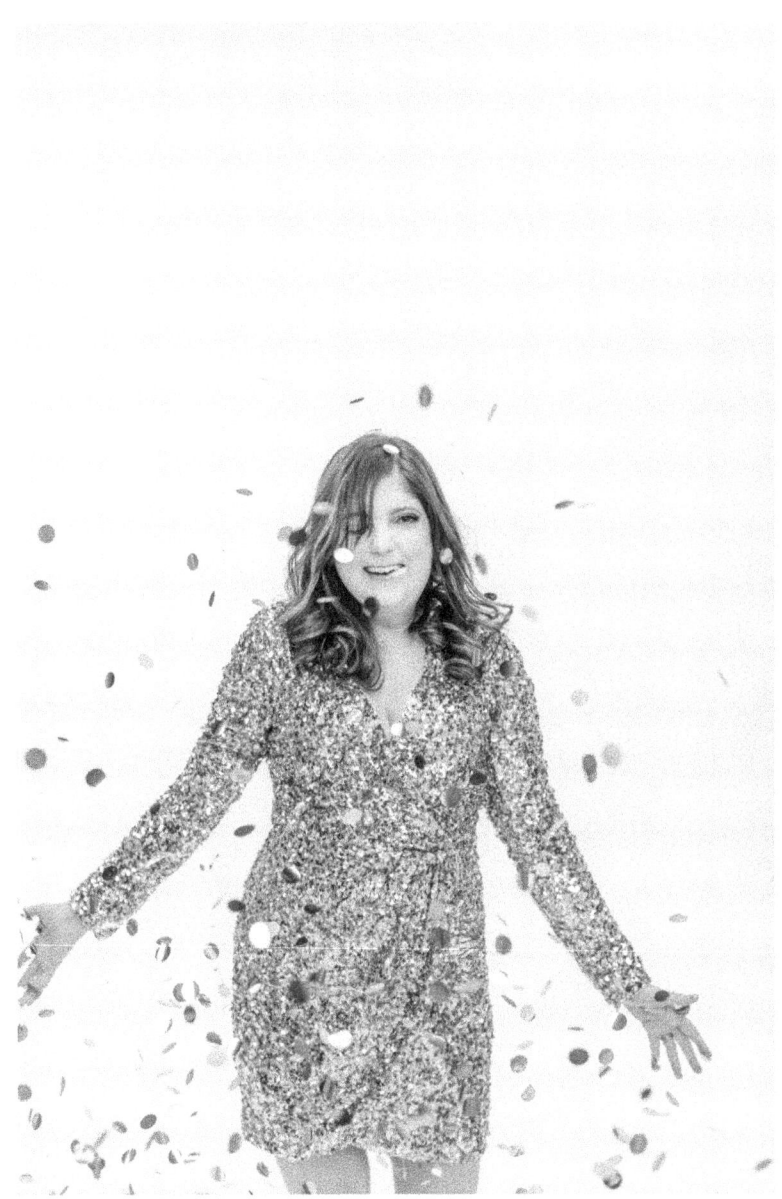

AFTERWORD

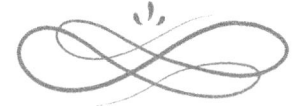

Well, I guess that brings us to 2023 and I can happily report that I have been hospital free since November 2022 and plan to keep it that way.

I have really spent time making sure I look after myself, nourishing my body with healthy foods, drinking plenty of water, exercising and ensuring that I listen to my body when it tells me to rest. As much as I don't want to! Oh, and I do have the sneaky fried hot chips and the occasional chocolate because you only live once and I do not believe you if you tell me you eat healthy 100% of the time.

No one wants to be friends with the 'sick' one; I have truly struggled with being around my friends and family as I feel like I have been treated differently. From time to time, I have felt like a burden on everyone around me. I feel people are unable to be themselves around me and are always very cautious.

Inspirational is a word used to describe the ability to feel something or do something creative.

Resilience is a word used to describe someone or something that has the capacity to recover quickly from a difficult situation.

Strong can be used to describe someone that can physically move a heavy object or can be strong minded.

Positive has so many different meanings but in my case, I have been known to have a positive mindset and that I am always expecting the good in every situation.

Vulnerable is being exposed to something that could harm you physically or mentally.

Friendly is to be kind and *honest* is to be truthful.

Generous is to give something to someone and to be *Grateful* is to appreciate something that you have received.

Survival is the skill to continue to live and push forward despite what comes your way.

Focus is to have a clear vision to achieve what you want by finding and having a solution.

To be *lucky* is to receive something good.

AFTERWORD

All of these descriptive words have been used to define me and I feel humble to know that people have used such beautiful words.

Although, I am simply Em, this is my story and I would feel honoured to be able to help anyone who is in a similar situation. I have been through more than what one person would go through in a lifetime but that does not make me better than anyone else. In any situation, there is always going to be something worse out there. Humanity provides lessons to others.

Everyone has always said that I am like a cat with nine lives but as you can see now that I have defied every odd up against me more than nine times. So I now I have upgraded to a phoenix!

I am always rising and creating a new cycle in life. I mean, I could always be a cockroach, not pleasant but you can't kill them, right?

I am also a professional or expert patient now and I do not want any sympathy but to simply motivate others. Grateful for my husband as some people would end their relationship if their partner was dealing with all of these medical issues.

Surprisingly, I have never experienced a mental health diagnosis and have the abilty to pull myself out of any bad situation. I always see the good in a situation.

Some of my quotes that I have created and kept me going that I would like to share with you all are:

"A smile happens in a flash but its memory lasts a lifetime."

"Life is a rollercoaster but you still come back smiling."

"Being positive doesn't mean that everything is good – it's the ability to see the good in everything."

I cannot wait to see what the future holds for me and where this opportunitity is going to take me and I look forward to sharing it all with you.

ABOUT THE AUTHOR

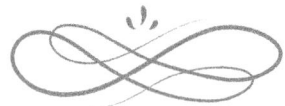

Emmilia has always wanted to write a book for as long as she can remember. When she first started dealing with her complex health challenges and surviving them, she knew she had to help people and younger people in similar situations to her. She did not want to go back to university and then work in a hospital that follows protocols, she wanted to share her experiences and support people in the hope that it will inspire others and she has now achieved that by writing her book.

Emmilia has endured more in her short thirty years on Earth than what one person would in their entire lifetime, however she has never let any health issue define her and strongly believes that she has lived a fulfilling life so far with so much more to come.

Emmilia lives with her husband, Aaron, in Doreen, Melbourne, Victoria, with their two blue heeler dogs, Skye & Banjo. Emmilia and Aaron have been together for thirteen years, since 2010, and have experienced everything good and bad life has to offer.

In Emmilia's spare time, she enjoys cooking wholesome tasty meals in her kitchen, spending time with her husband, family and friends, and taking her car for a drive.

Emmilia can not wait to meet and share her story with you.

Website: emmiliaosullivan.com
Email: emmilia@emmiliaosullivan.com
Facebook: Emmilia O'Sullivan
Instagram: @emmiliaosullivan
Tiktok: @emmiliaosullivan
Linked In: Emmilia O'Sullivan

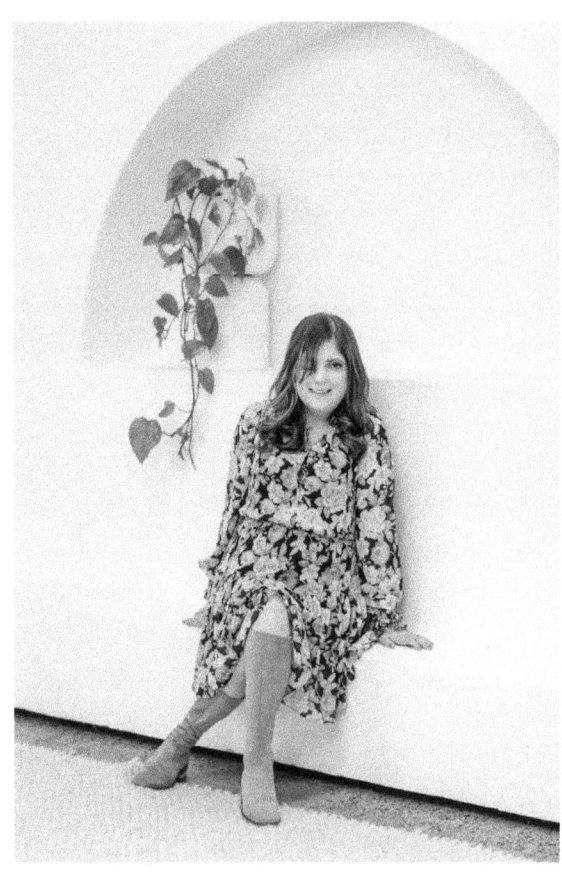

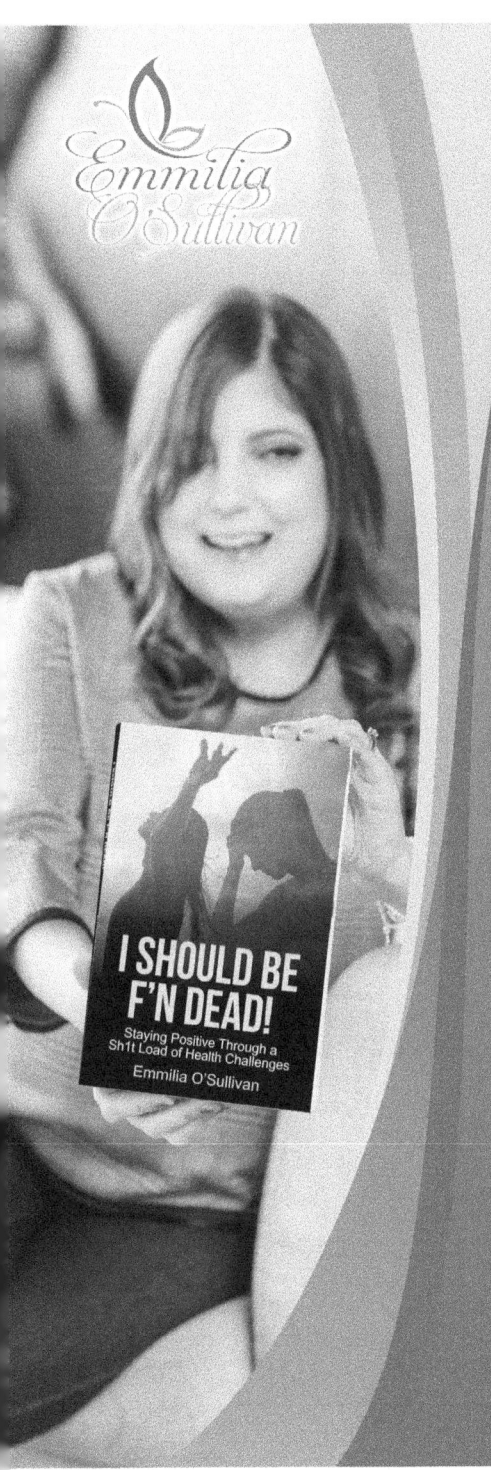

Emmilia O'Sullivan

is an inspirational young lady who has faced life's challenges head on and always does so with positivity and humour.

She is full of life, enthusiastic, and very passionate about providing support to people like her that have been through horrendous medical issues/diagnoses.

In Emmilia's short 30 years, she has endured more medical diagnoses' than one person would experience in their entire lifetime including Nephrectomy, Kidney Transplant, Spinal Fusion, Neck Dissections, Cardiac Arrest, Craniotomy, Non-Hodgkin's Lymphoma, Pneumonia, Sepsis and so much more!

She has defied all odds over and over again and is here to tell the tale. Emmilia wanted to write a book about her life in the hope to inspire others and show them you can come out great on the other end so that is exactly what she did and now shares her experiences with "I Should be F'N Dead!"

An open and approachable speaker, Emmilia shares all her experiences within the medical world with her audiences leaving them hopeful of the future and inspired to overcome any challenge they may face. Having someone that you can relate to gives a sense of comfort during the bad times and knowing that you are not alone truly helps. And as an added bonus, she may even make you laugh!

Emmilia is available to speak to support groups, events, organisations, schools and within the community. Her main topics are:

The Power of a Positive Mindset
- How to cope when receiving a life changing medical diagnoses
- Never giving up – The John Cena Way
- Celebrating the small wins

The Ultimate Recovery Conditions
- The keys to looking after yourself
- How to listen to your body
- Building the resilience muscle

Getting Up From Rock Bottom
- The power of practicing gratitude
- Finding your purpose
- Baby Steps for Big Outcomes

To enquire about engaging Emmilia to speak at your next event email
emmilia@emmiliaosullivan.com
to enquire about pricing and availability.

www.ingramcontent.com/pod-product-compliance
Lightning Source LLC
Chambersburg PA
CBHW041317110526
44591CB00021B/2820